Tony Hogan lived in Dublin and travelled all over Ireland as a highly acclaimed spiritual healer. He died in 2004.

BORN
TO HEAL

GUIDANCE AND INSIGHT FROM AN
EXTRAORDINARY IRISH HEALER

TONY HOGAN

RIDER

LONDON · SYDNEY · AUCKLAND · JOHANNESBURG

11

First published in 2002 by Rider, an imprint of Ebury Press, Random House, 20 Vauxhall Bridge Road, London SW1V 2SA

www.rbooks.co.uk

Addresses for companies within The Random House Group Limited can be found at: www.randomhouse.co.uk/offices.htm

The Random House Group Limited Reg. No. 954009 www.randomhouse.co.uk

A CIP catalogue record for this book is available from the British Library

The Random House Group Limited supports The Forest Stewardship Council (FSC), the leading international forest certification organisation. All our titles that are printed on Greenpeace approved FSC certified paper carry the FSC logo. Our paper procurement policy can be found at www.rbooks.co.uk/environment

Typeset by seagulls
Printed and bound in Great Britain by CPI Antony Rowe, Chippenham, Wiltshire

ISBN 9780712659468

CONTENTS

List of Exercises. vi
Acknowledgements vii

1 Born to Heal 1
2 Coming to Dublin. 14
3 It Never Rains, But It Pours. 37
4 The Healing Experience 60
5 Auras. 87
6 Healing Children 100
7 They Suffered in Silence 118
8 The Healing of Animals and Pets. 143
9 Healing the Impossible 151
10 Vitamin and Mineral Advice 170
11 Does Healing Always Work? 179
12 Absent Healing. 189
13 The Spirit World 210
14 The Gifts That We Have 220
15 You Can Heal Yourself 226

Bibliography 246

LIST OF EXERCISES

The Healing Breath. 86
Seeing Auras. 98
Healing for Your Child. 116
How to Ask for Help 141
How to Help Your Pet or Animal to Cope with a Journey . 149
How to Get Back in Touch with Yourself. 169
How to Compile a Diet History 178
How to Acknowledge Your Healing 187
Meditations –
   Enter the Silence and A Healing Prayer of Light 208
How to Communicate with Lost Loved Ones. 218
How to Discover Your Natural Gifts. 225
Breathe to Relax 227
How to Relax – the Method 228
Creative Visualisation –
   Using the Power of Your Mind to Heal Yourself 230
The Lemon Exercise 230
The Healing House. 233
The Healing Power of Music 236
Colour Healing 237
How to Control Pain 238
How to Stop Worrying. 238
Positive Affirmations 239
Laughter – The Best Medicine. 242
Write Out Your Problems. 243
How to Do Hands-on Healing 243
How to Do Absent Healing. 244

ACKNOWLEDGEMENTS

With Appreciation

This book would not have been written except for the help, support and kindness shown to me from the following people ...

To my mother Sarah; my family Billy, Patrick, Eileen and their families. Aunt Sis and Mary Walsh – love to you all.

A heartfelt thanks to Cathal Black, the gifted filmmaker, who believed in my work and who gave me the most wonderful support. Against all the odds he went out and made a film about my life, then pushed doors open for this book to be born. I am grateful also for his significant contribution to the shaping of the text – bless you.

To Moira O Broin for her relentless love, kindness and support shown to me down through the years – who told me to tell my story as it happened, and I did.

Thanks to my publisher Judith Kendra, my editor Susan Lascelles, and all at Random House for your wonderful work.

To Pam Buckley and all her family – thank you for your wonderful support and kindness shown to me all those years.

For Austin Byrne, the gifted astrologer, who has always given me great advice and encouragement, and who predicted this book a long time ago. I hope your stars always shine bright.

A warm thanks to Philip and Joy Ordman for their kindness and support shown to me over the years.

To my spirit friends who have guided me from the beginning.

To all my friends and patients, both past and present, who taught me so much and who trusted me. A warm thanks ...

This book is for you ...

I would like to thank sincerely all the people who told their stories, some of which came from an hour-long television documentary called 'The Invisible World – Portrait of an Irish Spiritual Healer'. Where necessary, names have been changed to protect their privacy.

CHAPTER 1

BORN TO HEAL

'A soul travels through the heavens,
and bursts like a star into being,
A new book of life opens ready to be written.
On the blank pages of the ether the cosmic pen begins to write,
As the first breath is taken the divine rejoice and sing.
The golden thread begins to weave as slowly time awakens,
The child on its path and the first step is taken.'

Tony Hogan

IF THEY HAD PUNCTURED the caul* and broken the waters before I was delivered, I probably would have died, they said. I had arrived into the world, weak and chronically ill; it was touch and go from the time I took my first breath. The doctor held me under running water to cool my roaring temperature. He warned my parents of possible blindness, crippling breathing problems and severe hearing loss. All would be accentuated as I grew older.

It was springtime in the mid 1950s in Dublin. The weather was

---

**A caul is the name given to the membrane covering the foetus; part of this covers the head of some infants at birth.*

warm for April, my mother recalled, and the cherry blossoms bloomed earlier than usual that year.

'Where in God's name have they put ye?' my father complained, through a mask over his face.

We had been quarantined in the hospital basement, isolated from the other patients. My father had to make his way down a tiled staircase, past the boiler room and laundry to find us. I had contracted German measles, so they christened me early.

Children died from it, the doctors said. There was no cure. It was up to me to survive. They kept us in the basement for weeks – my mother helpless and distressed as she saw me struggling to breathe, the nurses rushing me to the doctor whenever my temperature soared, the same doctor holding me naked under freezing cold tap water, leaving me to dry out on a table strewn with rubber sheeting.

When they finally allowed us home, the worry wasn't over. For three long months my mother brought me back and forth to the hospital for regular check-ups, she herself weak and debilitated from the stress and exhaustion of looking after me.

A wise old nurse, however, told my parents that they had a special child. The caul, she believed, had miraculously protected me and saved my life.

She'd seen a caul before, she said, around the baby's head moments after the birth – but this was different. I was enveloped from head to toe in its membrane, asleep and suspended in water, making my delivery extraordinarily peaceful and easy.

Old folk valued the caul's healing properties, the nurse said. They believed the caul could ward off sorcery and evil. Fishermen would buy a caul to protect them from drowning. A child born in one was uniquely talented, the old nurse explained. The child had the gift of healing, the power of second sight, even the ability to see ghosts. 'Your baby is rare and special,' she told my parents, as I screamed the place down.

A green Hillman, smoke billowing from its exhaust, trundles past luscious green fields and trees in full bloom. My mother holds me in her arms. My father sits in the front holding Billy, my older brother.

I'm the second to be born within two years. A kindly neighbour drives. My mother is wan and sickly. My birth combined with the German measles has left its mark.

My father, barely able to cope himself, is worried for us both. We are heading into County Wicklow, where my grandmother lives. She will take me in to live with her. I am barely four months old. But I will live with my grandmother for seven extraordinary years.

'Granny Brien', as I called her, was an impressive woman, strong and authoritative. A widow, she dressed entirely in black; wore black brogues, a black dress and a sweeping black shawl. Her hair was white – snow white against her black attire. It swept around her head where she tied it in a bun at the nape of her neck. She was the first real influence in my life and perhaps the biggest.

The most striking memory of those early years spent with my grandmother was the network of support and sharing that bound together the people in the community. Granny Brien was the hub of this network. She was the woman who knew how to cure ailments. She was the woman whom the local people came to talk to, if they were in trouble or had a problem. People came from near and far, young and old.

Once a nurse in the local hospital, Granny Brien still found time to visit the sick and dying in the community. Many suffered with tuberculosis and pneumonia, the common illnesses of the time.

I went with her everywhere, listening attentively to her every word. I remember she had two big silver candlesticks and, whenever she wrapped them carefully in a brown paper bag, I knew we were off to see someone who wasn't going to talk back to us.

Family, friends and neighbours would crowd in the hall and living room, waiting patiently for my grandmother to appear.

Without further ado, we'd head up the stairs to the bedroom of the deceased.

As Granny Brien prepared the person for burial, I'd catch a glimpse through an open door of her moving around the room, her sacred candlesticks burning in their silver holders, her voice strong and authoritative, even in a whisper – quietly instructing those around her. She had total respect for everyone – even the dead.

Downstairs, while I sat in a chair, with a biscuit and a glass of lemonade in hand, Granny Brien would comfort the heartbroken family, crying and grieving in their loss. I'd watch her chatting and laughing and telling stories about the good old days. And in no time at all – the atmosphere would lift and soon she had everyone in hysterics – breaking their sides laughing at her antics.

She was a tower of strength to everyone she came into contact with. Times were hard. All around us people were very poor; each day was a struggle. Many had left the countryside and cities of Ireland and taken the boat for England.

Some days we'd fill two bags with my grandmother's home-made soda bread, an apple tart, half-a-dozen eggs from the chickens she kept and jars of raspberry jam, and head off to visit a house a few miles away.

In we'd go for a few brief moments, then leave minus all the food – me running after Granny Brien as she strode purposefully back to our house; always busy, always caring, always giving with a good heart.

In wintertime, our life centred around the cosy log fire. At night the fire threw shadows dancing across the walls and ceiling. We slept downstairs in the front room; yellow light spilling through the open door from the old gas lamp, that shimmered above the fireplace in the living room. The hall door was always open; sick and grieving people arriving at all hours of the day and night. My job was to put the kettle on for tea, while they sat around the fire and told stories of their sadness and heartache.

Granny Brien would listen intently, taking in their every word, consoling them in their upset. Advice would be given – eyes would brighten and when it was time to leave, they always felt the better for coming. A burden shared, a load lifted.

I remember the old grandfather clock ticked away on the mantelpiece above the fire. Granny Brien sat on her rocking chair on one side – me on the other. With knitting needles in her hands and a great big ball of wool on her lap, she'd tell me stories about her life – bursting into fits of belly laughter as the memories came – sending the ball of brightly coloured wool flying across the room.

The silence was only broken by footsteps in the hall. The handle of the door turning – 'It's only me!' a voice would call from the darkness.

'Who's me?' Granny Brien would enquire mischievously. A great big shadow running up the wall as the figure entered the room.

'Me! Ginny Murray.'

'Welcome, Ginny Murray. Come in and sit yourself down. Would you like a cup of tea or a glass of porter?'

'I'll have a sup,' was always Ginny's reply as she sat down by the blazing fire.

A few minutes passing, then more footsteps in the hall.

'It's only me! Essie,' and the handle of the door would turn. Granny Brien always made everyone welcome.

'Sit down beside the fire and get the heat into you. Throw your shawl there on the nail at the back of the door.'

Soon they were off into a world of conversation and laughter, swapping one funny story after another, while sipping on black porter. I'd sit in the rocking chair looking on, absorbed by the bright colours of the fire. Lost in my own little world and the invisible friends that peopled it. Our small living room was full of laughter and song, spilling on into the wee hours of the morning. In Granny Brien's world, time always stood still.

My grandmother regarded me as a special child with special gifts and told me this often. I spent a great deal of time listening to her wisdom. In a quiet moment she'd talk to me about my future; about the unusual job I'd be doing when I grew up. She knew I could see coloured light around people from an early age.

At night, when everything was quiet, I'd match the colours in the fire with people from the village; the passing nuns in the street – light blue, the shopkeeper – yellow. My grandmother would just listen and accept. To her it was just natural.

My parents came to visit whenever they could. It was a time of getting to know me a little better – giving me presents at Christmas.

'He's still pale and washed-out looking,' I'd hear them whisper.

'I'll hold on to him for a little longer,' my grandmother would say, smiling over at me as I hid under the table. However, when they left it was back to the old routine.

On Saturday nights, we'd find ourselves in the snug of the local pub crammed with women of Granny Brien's vintage. A box of snuff passed from table to table; a sniff and the women's noses looked peppered. Some smoked long clay pipes. I was convinced that they carried their fireplaces around with them, for heat.

Glasses empty – a woman would turn to me and cackle, 'Go up there son and give that wee door a good bang.' I'd wait for Granny Brien's approval.

A nod from her and I'd rap the door with my knuckles. 'That's a good boy,' one of the women would say as they carried on with their conversation. The hatch door would eventually slide open – a man's face poking out to look gruffly down on me. 'Six more glasses of porter and a glass of lemonade for the wee boy.' The man slammed the hatch door shut as he went to take the order.

Soon we were off on our journey home, bottles of porter wrapped up in a brown paper bag.

Granny Brien would stoke up the fire and put more logs on, and thrust her 'magic' poker into the hot ashes.

She'd pour porter into a glass, then scoop the red hot poker from the fire, ashes and all, and plunge it into the black stuff, the porter hissing with smoke wafting across the room.

'There you go, little one,' she'd say, handing me a small drop of her magic porter in a glass. 'It's an iron tonic; it'll help build you up for the winter.'

I still remember the bitter taste of that porter. Granny Brien would fall around the place laughing at the faces I pulled while trying to get down a few sups of her tonic.

Granny Brien had a cure for everything; special chicken broth and poultices for the sick. She'd make them up whenever I had a sty in my eye, or an abscess in the ear, or a toothache. Some were made of bread and boiling water, others were of dock leaf or a hot potato taken from the fire; all very effective in drawing out the poison.

Then there were her tonics: young wild nettles, water from a special well, wild berries, cabbage or onion tonic, seaweed for cuts and bruises, honey for sore throats and burns.

I was always looking over her shoulder, full of curiosity, as she made up her potions each night. But one day my curiosity got the better of me.

While Granny Brien was outside talking to a few neighbours, I picked up her oval-shaped silver snuff box. Why did all these women put that queer stuff up their noses, I wondered.

I carefully opened the small silver box and put a pinch of snuff on the back of my hand, then held my nose close by, shutting one nostril while sniffing hard with the other. With that, the stuff went right up my nose and immediately I went into a fierce bout of uncontrolled sneezing; dropping the snuff box on to the floor, scattering the precious powder everywhere.

In walked Granny Brien with some of the neighbours when she heard the commotion. I couldn't stop myself sneezing – tears rolling down my face. The more I sneezed the more they laughed, until a crowd of women and children were all gathered in the living room, breaking their sides laughing at my antics.

I learned a hard lesson that day, to stay away from that queer 'snuff stuff'.

Granny Brien loved going to see films, or 'the pictures', as she called them.

Her great big black shawl came in handy on these occasions. 'Get under my shawl, little one, and don't come out till I tell you,' she'd say as we approached the cinema.

'Now walk with me, when I walk,' she'd whisper, her hand firmly on my shoulder as she guided me along in a tomb of darkness. As soon as we were through the cinema door, out I'd come from beneath her shawl, into flashing lights and the roar of gunfire, just as the film started – her timing was always perfect.

People would leave clothes and children's toys at our house for the poor. Granny Brien would lay them in neat piles on the kitchen floor. Then we'd bundle them into separate bags, and off we'd go on our travels – dropping off children's clothes, scarves, gloves, overcoats, socks, blankets, a few toys, a teddy bear or a doll to a home in need. 'God bless you,' they'd say as we skipped from door to door, before it fell dark.

There were times when I found it hard to part with a teddy bear or a toy gun, while running after my gran.

But as soon as we went into a house, she'd say, 'Leave it there on the woman's table. The children need it, that's a good boy.'

Every day she cleaned houses, fed hungry children, went on errands for the sick and generally took time to provide every possible comfort for those in need of warmth and love. Whenever I saw her cooking for those who couldn't fend for themselves, instructing families on how to care for their sick parents or nursing me through my illnesses, I wanted to be like her.

At night she'd throw her big black shawl over the bed to keep us warm, then kneeling on the floor she'd pray aloud for those who were sick or in trouble. Bursting her sides laughing at something that had happened that day, she'd turn to me and say, 'We'll be a long time dead, little one. We'll be a long time dead.'

My Uncle Christy and Aunt Sis lived upstairs – son and daughter of Granny Brien. Both were out working all day and didn't encroach on our world.

I remember one cold winter's day, I was sitting up to the fire on the rocking chair. Granny Brien was in the kitchen making tea. There was a sudden waft of cold air as the front door opened.

Uncle Christy hurried in from work and, reaching into his inside pocket, took out a beautiful snow-white kitten and put her on the ground. She teetered on her legs for a moment, then walked over to me and crawled up into my lap. That night the kitten slept on top of Granny Brien's big black shawl close to me. The next morning I awoke to find a thick blanket of white powdery snow outside the window. It was the first time I'd seen snow. 'The kitten is the same as the snow,' I cried. From that moment on we called the kitten 'Snowball'.

When Snowball got a bit older, Granny Brien put a piece of red ribbon and a little silver bell around her neck.

Everywhere we went, Snowball walked behind us, her bell ringing. I had found a friend. She was the subject of much conversation throughout the community.

'Come quick, hurry!' a neighbour screamed as she burst through our front door. 'Nellie has passed out on the kitchen floor!'

Granny Brien instructed me to stay, and raced out the door after the neighbour.

Immediately I went into the bedroom to the mantelpiece where she had her two big candlesticks and got them ready. But within a few minutes she returned with the local bully Jimmy, Nellie's son – his face and clothes all covered in blood. He was twice my age and twice my height and as broad as a door. My stomach churned when I saw him. Jimmy was always in fights and I had some near misses with him when going to the shops for messages. But now blood was pouring down his face and dripping on to Granny Brien's clean linoleum floor.

'Leave him with me and go back and keep an eye on his mother,' Granny Brien instructed the neighbour – Nellie had fainted when she saw her son covered in blood.

'Sit down there, Jimmy,' Granny Brien urged as she held a big white towel to his face.

'Quick, little one – fetch me a porter bottle from under the sink, and fill it up with cold water,' Granny Brien instructed. Poor Snowball went scampering under the table as I ran to the kitchen.

Granny Brien put Jimmy lying flat down on the floor and placed the cold porter bottle under the nape of his neck.

'Stay there until I tell you to move,' she warned.

What a sight to behold! Here was Jimmy the local bully, who everyone was afraid of, lying across Granny Brien's kitchen floor, looking terrified. We mopped up the mess and tidied around. Soon all the stillness and peace came back into the room.

'How did it happen?' asked Granny Brien, as she sat Jimmy up on her chair beside the fire. Jimmy looked terribly shaken and sat with his head in his lap.

Granny Brien gave him tea and brack while she waited for his explanation. Slowly, he put his hand into his jacket pocket and took out a silver mouth organ.

'I was up the town – playing me mouth organ,' he said as he put it into his mouth and blew a few notes.

'I must of been playing it for too long – for me mouth started to bleed,' he said feebly.

Granny Brien took one look at me; the same withering look I'd seen so often when someone was in for a good telling off. Turning to Jimmy, she stared deep into his eyes and said flatly, 'You must've been playing your mouth organ up your nose!'

There was complete silence for a moment. Jimmy looked red-faced. Then suddenly, unable to contain myself any longer, I burst out laughing at the vision of Jimmy playing his mouth organ up his nose. Granny Brien also exploded with laughter, filling the whole room with her presence.

'For as long as I know you Jimmy; and that's since you were in a pram, you were always fighting. You were always in trouble.'

Jimmy's head went down into his lap. 'Please don't tell me mother what happened. Please don't,' he begged.

Granny Brien lifted his chin and stared into his frightened face and said, 'I am not your mother, Jimmy, and don't ever come in here telling your lies to me.'

Pointing her finger at me, she followed with – 'Furthermore, if I ever catch you laying a finger on that boy there, you will have more than a bloody nose.'

Jimmy's head sunk further into his chest. He shook with fear and started crying. Granny Brien must have known all along the threat that Jimmy had put me under.

From that day on everyone remarked on the complete change that had come over Jimmy. He knocked on our door early each morning, wondering if we wanted anything done.

Granny Brien made him ask the old people if they needed any errands from the shop. Sometimes, Jimmy would borrow a wheelbarrow and take me off to places I had never been before; fetching turf and logs for Granny Brien and her neighbours. He'd put me sitting in between the sacks of turf and wheel me all the way home; playing his mouth organ and singing aloud, 'I wheeled my wheel barrow, through streets broad and narrow, singing cockles and mussels alive, alive O.'

If any of Jimmy's gang started picking on me he would refer to me as his little brother, and quickly they'd back off. It was Granny Brien that made him change. She saw the good in people and always brought out the best in them.

I lived simultaneously in a world of sickness and pain, and in a world of healing. My grandmother's ability to comfort people, to make them well again, left a deep and lasting impression on me. As time went on I learned to appreciate and value the many gifts she had.

One day, while running to answer her call to dinner, I fell and cut my knees on some stony gravel outside the house. A neighbour tried to get me to stand but I felt completely numb.

Try as I might, my legs wouldn't move. My two kneecaps looked as if they had come clean off. I fell back on the road and cried from the terrible shooting pains and the sight of blood pouring down my legs. Out of the house came my grandmother; cool as a cucumber. She didn't ask whether I could walk – instinctively she knew I couldn't.

As I sat there in agony with the pain, Granny Brien stooped down on the road beside me and put her two hands gently on my knees. Immediately, I felt a tingling sensation. It was coming from her hands; a sensation both soothing and comforting. Suddenly, the blood stopped running from my knees. The pain eased.

Granny Brien looked deep into my eyes and said, 'You're all right little one. Up you come.' I stood as if on a cushion of air and walked across the small roadway into the house. Terrified to look down at my knees, I sat on the chair and had my dinner. When I'd finished eating, I walked to the kitchen sink to wash my hands. Without thinking, I looked down; my knees were completely better. I couldn't believe it! How did she do that? – I wondered.

For days afterwards I'd check my knees to see if they were still intact. My grandmother would catch me looking and burst out laughing at my puzzlement. To me, Granny Brien was magic; she had magic hands.

Little did I realise then that this experience, firmly stamped within my inner mind, was a clear indication of my future work as a healer.

One day I fell into a light sleep; I could hear my grandmother moving quietly around the room. I opened my eyes and looked at her. The light around her was waning. Immediately, I became very upset and cried out, 'Gran, you're not there. You're gone!'

'What's wrong, little one?' she asked, as she tried her best to soothe me.

'You're gone, you're not there You're gone!' I cried again. Granny Brien understood as always; she knew that I was frightened; that I'd seen something that had upset me deeply. Quietly, softly she comforted me; reassuring me over and over that everything would be all right.

A few weeks later, at the great age of eighty-six, Granny Brien passed away.

She was laid out in her bedroom with her two beautiful silver candlesticks burning brightly above her bed, the same ones she used to light up so many other people's rooms. Crowds came from everywhere to pay their respects and to tell their stories of how much she helped them. She gave her heart and her love to everyone.

My whole world turned upside down.

CHAPTER 2

COMING TO DUBLIN

'Hands of invisible spirits touch the strings of that mysterious instrument, the soul, and play the prelude of our future.'
Henry Wadsworth Longfellow

I WAS SEVEN YEARS OLD when I left Wicklow and went on the big green bus to the capital city. My mother and father had come to get me – to bring me to Dublin for a short holiday. They told me stories of how wonderful it was going to be.

Their house was one of two red-brick cottages, nestling off a lane-way in Rathmines. A beautiful lilac tree, full of blossoms and perfume, hung over the side wall.

When my father turned the key in the door, a feeling of apprehension came over me; I was frightened of this new life and yearned for the one I'd left behind. I stepped inside and saw a turf fire blazing and the table set.

My mother went to the kitchen to prepare some food. Billy, my older brother, would be along later, they said, after his game of football.

As we ate I looked across the table at these strange people – was this to be my new home?

The front door was cut in half and there was no upstairs. I'd seen many a door like this in the country, but horses lived there – was I going to live in a stable, I wondered.

When my father unlocked the back door, three golden-haired spaniels, Kim, Paddy and Fritz, crashed into the room and leapt all over me. I fell madly in love with them all, and as the days progressed I spent endless hours chasing them around the back garden.

Soon the novelty of the holiday wore off. I needed to escape. But the half-door prevented me from returning home. Every day I tried to climb over the door to return to Wicklow. My grand-mother was waiting for me there, I cried.

The more I pulled at the door, the more my breathing gave way. Finally, I collapsed from exhaustion. My parents tried to comfort me as best they could during these troubled times, but I was inconsolable.

Dublin was a different world for me. Poor people lived in large tenements – I marvelled at how they all crammed together in one big house. Instinctively I felt sorry for them. The old women dressed in black, just like my grandmother, and sat on doorsteps watching malnourished children playing barefoot in the streets.

Every street registered a distinct feeling within me – unusual light and colours and odours that lingered in the air.

'Son, you can tell where you are in Dublin by the smell,' my father would say, 'just follow your nose!'

There was the Guinness brewery smell, the Jacob's biscuit factory smell. Bolands bread mills, and the horrible smell of the River Liffey.

'You'll have to get to know your bearings around here son – otherwise you'll get lost. Then where would we be?' my father impressed upon me, clutching my hand tightly.

Walking through streets of cobbled stones across the old iron tram-tracks and over the canal bridge in Rathmines, my father would point to where George Bernard Shaw once lived.

James Joyce had lived on the road at the back of our house; a spot on the ground in Moore Street was where a famous Irish republican got shot.

'Willie! Willie, come here,' a familiar voice shouted over the traffic noise in Grafton Street. It was 'the Bold Brendan Behan,' as my father called him.

'Come for a drink Willie,' Behan would insist. And with a few coppers pressed into my hand, we were off to McDaid's pub for the afternoon.

On our way home I was sworn to secrecy about where we'd been, especially if my mother asked.

In upper Rathmines we'd meet 'Mixer Reid', the dwarf. His adult voice and crinkled face scared me. He'd stand on the street corner talking to my father, and place the flat of his hand on my head. As he measured his height with mine, I could feel his hand on my skin, dry as parchment.

Another character we'd meet at night was the famous actor, Micheal Mac Liammoir. He was always dressed in a long black cloak with white stuff on his face.

'Just come off the stage, Micheal?'

'Full house! Willie! Full house!' he'd shout, his voice booming as he sailed home through the fog of Harcourt Street.

Horses and carts were common on the streets of Dublin. Sometimes I'd play with the horses as they drank from decorative stone water troughs, my father chatting and smoking with the owner. We'd take regular walks from Portobello Bridge, along the canal down to Baggot Street where my father delivered books to Parsons, the bookshop.

There was always a man there I recall, pacing up and down the canal bank, muttering to himself.

'Da – why is that man talking to himself?'

'That's Paddy Kavanagh, the poet, son,' my father explained.

'What's a poet, Da? Does it make you talk to yourself?'

'You'll learn all about it when you go to school, son.'

The summer months were coming to an end, the days getting shorter. I was out playing with the dogs in the back garden when my father came out to talk to me.

'You know, being at home all the time playing with the dogs is not the best situation for you son,' he cajoled.

'How would you like to go to school with your brother, Billy?'

From that moment on I knew the holidays were over.

A heavy iron green gate opened into an austere red-brick building on the main Rathmines Road. 'Built in 1823', a grey stone plaque declared.

The girls' part of the school was to the right, the boys' part to the left. The tiny yard was littered with broken glass. Heavy wired cages covered the school windows.

The surrounding walls were very high and frightening looking. I'd never seen such a place before in my life.

We climbed a long wooden staircase. My mother knocked on the glass door; I could hear children reciting from the corridor. Mrs Nolan, the principal, stepped out from her classroom and stared at me with piercing blue eyes. My mother explained that my brother Billy had already been through her hands.

'What's your name?' she snapped.

My mind went blank. I looked away. Mrs Nolan had flaming red curly hair and a temper to match.

'Hogan,' replied my mother for me.

Who were they talking about? I wondered. My name was Brien – as in Granny Brien.

'Look at me when I'm talking to you!' Mrs Nolan hissed.

I froze. Nobody had ever spoken to me like this before.

'What's two and two?' she barked, and stooped to get a good look at me.

'What's three and three?'

When I didn't answer, Mrs Nolan peered at me with disdain.

'He's very backward, isn't he?' she stated flatly.

'What age is he now?'

'He's just gone seven years, Mrs Nolan.'

'SEVEN!' Mrs Nolan screeched. 'Why wasn't he in school before this?'

My mother explained about my poor health. About living with my grandmother.

'Wasn't his grandmother aware he should have been in school a long time ago?' she asked suspiciously.

I smiled at the thought of Granny Brien not knowing something.

If Mrs Nolan only knew Granny Brien, I said to myself, as my mind drifted back to a world that felt safe and to the people who had accepted me for what I was.

Mrs Nolan finally told my mother she hadn't any room in her school. She would write in due course if a place became available.

Relived to get away from that strange lady, I started walking backwards on the footpath through the autumn leaves, mimicking what Mrs Nolan had said about me.

'What's backward. What did she mean I was backward?' I asked my mother repeatedly.

'Mind yourself son, or you'll fall over. Turn around, like a good boy.'

'But what's backward?' I kept asking – pressing my mother for an answer.

'Oh, ask your father when you get home,' she chuckled.

Not long afterwards I started school.

'Come with me,' Mrs Nolan snapped, clicking her fingers as she went. I followed her downstairs to a classroom in the basement, my shoes squeaking on the polished floor.

Mrs Nolan had a word with the teacher and put me sitting

beside a young child, in a room full of small children. I sat looking down on them – my two big knees sticking out of the desk.

They called me 'The Giant,' and laughed hysterically when I came crashing off the seat on to the floor.

The teacher wasn't amused. I was quickly frog-marched up the stairs to Mrs Nolan. After a lot of whispering and odd looks, she told me to sit in a desk more my size.

Introducing me as 'the new boy who'd come up from the country,' Mrs Nolan made it perfectly clear that I had a lot of catching up to do if I was to stay in her school. I vividly remember seeing a deep red colour, flashing and flaring around her head, whenever we didn't know the answers to her questions.

During the winter I became quite ill with my breathing, and spent more and more time at home in bed. My brother Billy reckoned I had a great thing going – staying at home all day with my mother and the three dogs. By the time I was ready to return to school, I found myself in a new class. I had graduated to the boys' school, and to the harsh brutality meted out by the male teachers. In time I got better at reading and writing, gradually awakening to what school life was all about.

My parents lived a simple life. We had no clock in our house, but the town hall rang on the half-hour, telling us the time. The big moon-faced clock could be seen clearly from our lilac tree. Every morning, Billy or I would be sent out to see what time it was. I could only report what the big hand was doing, and what the little hand was up to. Many is the time I'd get the two hands mixed up, and have the whole house late.

When winter's frost was thick on the ground, I'd skate up to the corner to look down the lane at the clock.

But with fog or mist lying about it was almost impossible to see. Billy and I would be dispatched to see if either of us could make out the correct time – with many arguments as to who was right.

When spring came around, we'd spend many an hour playing

high up in the branches of the lilac tree, listening to the lazy conversations of those who passed below. In summer, the lilac's perfume hung in the warm air.

Our neighbours would stop under the canopy of blossoms and breathe in its sweet scent – unaware that I was camouflaged high up in its branches, looking down in amusement as the colours around them brightened and expanded.

I had spent my early years among women, with Granny Brien and her friends. Now, life was peopled with odd families and even more curious men. There was the poor family that lived in an old green bus down the lane, with no running water or electricity, and rags hanging on the windows for curtains.

There was 'Barney Rubble' who had a bubble car. Every night, Barney and my Da would lift the little three-wheeler over the wall into Barney's back garden, throw a big foxford blanket across its body to protect it from the frosty nights and lift it out again the following morning. There was Mr Brenner, the German pilot who was captured during the war and who lived alone in a small galvanised shed. He never spoke to us kids, but banged all day long with his hammer, moulding steel rubbish bins that he sold on the street. In the evenings, I could hear him talking in a stammer in broken English to my father while we played football in the lane – squeezing out the last drops of time before the call for bed.

Winter came. Overnight, a blanket of pure white snow covered the gardens and rooftops. I peeped out from under the bedclothes, and my mind wandered back to the day Snowball, the kitten, arrived at Granny Brien's house.

I remembered the way the snow fell magically the next morning, and how I'd named her Snowball, on seeing the snow. It was a fairyland I wanted to return to for ever. But alas, these happy moments were overshadowed by the harsh reality of school.

It was time for hearing and eye tests. Time to have our weight checked and our teeth examined. Something was up, I feared, because the nurse kept calling me back for more tests. Finally, a note was dispatched home to my parents.

My father told me I didn't have to go to school the following day – we'd go into town on the bus instead he said.

I clung tightly to my father's arm as we reached a grey, forbidding building in town. A strange feeling engulfed me; a feeling I'd felt before when I was in danger. Little did I realise that this was the Corn Market Dental Hospital. A shiver ran up my spine as I passed through the great oak doors into an empty hallway.

Up the marble staircase we went, my legs heavy as lead. The dreadful smell of gas was everywhere.

'What's that smell?' I asked my father in a whisper.

When we reached the top of the stairs I saw two people standing at the end of a long dark corridor, smiling at me. A strange light surrounded them. They seemed so far away, yet so near. We sat on a big black leather sofa facing an open door. Beyond the door, dappled sunlight poured through a large Victorian window. Next to the open door, another door opened. A man in a white coat came out and whispered something into my father's ear, barely glancing at me as he disappeared again through the same door.

My father looked at me and said, 'You see through that open door, son? You see that chair? I want you to go and sit on that chair. It'll be like the barber's where you get your hair cut. I'll be there in a minute. I just want to talk to the man that was here a moment ago. Go on now, go!' he urged.

I stepped slowly towards the door, glancing back at my father – and at the two people radiating light who were standing at the end of the corridor, still smiling at me.

I saw the black leather chair and went towards it. My father waved me on. As I climbed into the chair the door suddenly banged shut. My head snapped around. The man in the white coat came from behind and grabbed my arms tightly. Four more people in white coats ran in, grabbed my legs and pinned me down. I bucked and kicked with as much force as I could muster. Two went flying backwards against a window – a loud thump as one head hit the glass.

'Quick! Grab his feet!' another shouted.

Two came from behind and pinned my arms down, while a third forced a mask over my head. The two who had hit the window recovered quickly and held me down. I struggled and screamed.

While all this commotion was going on, my eyes were firmly fixed on the couple who stood across the room to my left; the same couple I'd seen earlier in the corridor.

Suddenly, everything went into slow motion. Faintly I heard a voice say, 'I think we have him now.' I struggled one last time but I'd lost all the fight left within me. The room began to spin. Distantly I heard another voice say, 'It's all right, little one! It's all right.'

It was a voice I would recognise anywhere – it was the voice of Granny Brien. She was standing on my left, with the same couple who kept smiling at me.

I stepped down off the chair, my eyes riveted on Granny Brien. 'Come here little one, you are all right,' she beckoned and opened her arms wide. I ran straight into her loving arms, and felt her peace fill me with boundless love and comfort.

Glancing back across the room, I saw a little boy lying on the chair, surrounded by all these big people. And felt a great sadness for him.

'Come with me,' Granny Brien whispered, and when I turned to her, she held out her big warm hand, and we went through a doorway of mist, into a beautiful place in the country. The grass was deep green and vibrant. The birds spoke a language I under-stood. A sparkling river flowed by a white-washed cottage. It was the most beautiful place I had ever seen. This was a place where Granny Brien lived and loved. I wanted to stay with her for ever. But alas, 'It's time to go back, little one,' she said.

She held my hand tightly and we were back in the room once again. The same couple were there smiling at me – as if to say, 'You're back!' I could see the little boy being wheeled out of the room by the man in a white coat.

Granny Brien whispered, 'It's all right, little one. You have nothing to fear,' and she kissed me gently on the forehead. 'I'm here. I'm always here if you ever need me.'

I felt a sudden rush, like water rushing down a plug hole and awoke in another room with my head over a sink, spitting blood.

'Are you all right, son? Are you all right?' I heard my father say.

I slowly came to. Stark white hand-basins lined the walls. I looked over my father's shoulder. The same two lighted people that I'd seen with Granny Brien were standing close by. They smiled, one last time, before vanishing into a grey-white mist. My father turned to see what I was looking at, 'There's nobody there, son,' he said.

That afternoon I came home minus thirteen teeth, but clinging to the wonderful experience I'd had with my Granny Brien.

Many strange and wonderful characters lived in our neighbourhood. But there was one man I felt was very different from all the others.

'Michael's Shop' was at the other end of our lane. I'd pass by the little grocery shop as I went to and from school.

Whenever I had a few pence, I'd go in, unscrew the black lids on the jars and take out two black toffees, a few bull's-eyes or a penny fizz-bag. Each time, a voice bellowed from the darkness, 'Put the money on the counter, son. Just leave it there and go away.'

Cigarette smoke curled up from Michael's hand as he sat in darkness at the end of the counter. I only heard his voice, never saw him close up.

But one day my curiosity overpowered me. I tiptoed into his shop, taking each step slowly and quietly. Holding on to the long wooden counter, I came face to face with Michael. He sat fast asleep on his high stool. I noticed that his fingers were very long; his nails spotlessly clean. Ashes from his cigarette dropped slowly on to the counter top. Suddenly his head rose and fell. Terror and fear grabbed the pit of my stomach. I could see Michael's face now; he had thick black curly hair, streaked with Brylcreme.

My fear soon changed to sadness as I looked up into his child-like face and thought – what happened to this poor man? Why was he all dressed up in a black suit? With funny coat-tails hanging over the high stool?

Why was he wearing a red-spotted dicky bow? What was the white stuff on his face?

Michael let out a deep moan and the fear returned to the pit of my stomach. A dryness gripped my throat. I panicked. What would I say to him if he woke up?

Slowly, I retraced my steps back across the stone floor, reaching the safety of the counter. Just as I got to the door – Michael woke up.

'Who's there? Who ...?' he muttered.

'It's only me Michael, it's me.' I blurted out, speaking his name for the very first time. 'I just want ... some ... some sweets.'

There was a long, tense pause. Michael whined and then shouted back, 'Just take them son and get out.'

I quickly unscrewed the jar lid, my hands shaking as I took out twopence worth of sweets, dropped the money on the counter and ran.

Michael's home sat alongside his shop. Early on Sunday mornings when everyone was having a lie in, I'd find myself sitting on the footpath in the blazing sun, listening to the beautiful piano music that came through Michael's window. 'Where's that lovely music coming from?' people asked on their way to Mass. I always assumed that Michael had his radio turned on.

One day, while out on our rambles, I got my opportunity to question my father about Michael.

'It's a long story son,' he'd say. 'You're far too young to understand.'

'Oh, Da! Please tell me anyway,' I pressed.

'Why is Michael so different? He dresses oddly, where's his family?'

My father knew I wouldn't be fobbed off so easily.

We had just walked through the gates of Palmerston Park and eventually he gave in and said, 'When Michael was a young boy like yourself, he was a great pianist. In other words he played the piano.'

We stopped walking and sat down on a park bench. In anticipation of my next question, my father quickly continued, 'And when he grew up, his mother and father wanted him to become a doctor; so he was sent to university and then on to the College of Surgeons. You know the big building opposite St Stephen's Green?'

'Yes, yes!' I said impatiently.

'Well, Michael had only a few months to go before he qualified as a doctor. But then he had a nervous breakdown. This means he was very sick and they put him into hospital. In the mean time, his parents died and left him the house and the shop. When Michael eventually came out of the hospital, he stayed on there on his own, playing his grand piano. He never ventured outside the door after that.'

As we thought about Michael's sad life we fell silent for a few minutes; a deep silence broken only by the birds whistling and the wind rustling through the trees.

'That's the story about Michael, son. Follow your star, always follow your star. Remember that, son,' said my father, his voice faltering. I could see tears welling up in his eyes.

Something had struck a chord deep within me and I felt a terrible sadness for Michael.

'Come,' my father said briskly. 'We'll go and see Michael now, I want to get a few things for the tea tonight.'

As we walked along Palmerston Road to Michael's shop I continued to ask my father more questions, 'Do you know Michael well?'

'Yes of course I do. I grew up with him; he's a very kind, sensitive man. Don't ever be afraid of Michael, son. He has a heart of gold,' my father said as we crossed the road to the little shop.

'Ah! Willie it's you,' Michael said warmly, as he got off his stool and extinguished his cigarette. It was the first time I'd ever seen him rise for anyone – out of his tomb of darkness and into the light that beamed through the door.

'Is this your young boy, Willie?'

'This is him. Straight from his grandmother's arms in Wicklow,' my father said proudly.

'He's a lovely boy,' Michael said as he patted me on the head. 'There son, go over there and take some sweets from the jar – go on,' he insisted as he and my father chatted about the good old days – sometimes bursting into a bar of a song.

My father had a wonderful knack of bringing people out of themselves and as I chewed on a toffee sweet, I could see Michael light up inside.

'How would you like to come into the shop son, after school, and help me serve?' Michael asked suddenly.

'Yes! I'd love to!' I shouted and leaped into the air with the prospects of serving all the fellas on the road.

The next day I couldn't wait for half-past two to finish school. I ran all the way home, threw my school bag on the floor and raced up the road to stand behind the counter.

People came and went all afternoon; I served them bread, butter, milk, cigarettes and sweets to the children. Michael sat on his favourite stool in complete darkness, smoking his cigarette – his head drooping as he nodded off to sleep.

One particular Saturday, he turned to me and said, 'Will you get that brown cloth sack and put all the money into it from the big drawer. Go out the back – through the door on the left, lift the lid on the piano and leave it there. That's a good boy.'

I entered his house, dragging the heavy sack of money along the floor. Dusty sunlight streamed through the windows across the bleached furniture. The atmosphere was peaceful and still. I found myself stepping back in time.

A faded photograph of Michael's mother and father hung on the wall over the mantelpiece. Each room had a magnificent piano, sitting quietly in the shadows.

I remembered what my father had said about Michael, and the heavenly music I'd heard coming from his shop on Sunday mornings.

There were six pianos in all. When I lifted the lids, they were all chock-a-block with sacks of money. Where could I leave this new sack, I wondered.

I dragged the sack along the ground as far as I could – then returned to the shop to ask Michael which piano should I put it into, but found him fast asleep on his stool, snoring. I hauled the sack back into one of the rooms and left it up against the door of a wardrobe.

The clock on the wall struck half-past three. I started to close up the shop, while trying to make as little noise as possible. 'Did you do that, son?' Michael asked suddenly from his sleep.

'Yes Michael, I left it beside the wardrobe.'

'Ah, that's a good lad. I'm going to have me dinner now. If you sweep the floor and take something for yourself and lock the door after you, I'll see you on Monday. Tell your Da and Ma I was asking for them.'

As I swept the floor, the door into his house closed with a bang. A few minutes later, the most beautiful music came through the walls.

When I wasn't working in Michael's shop, I was off with the lads up 'the plots', picking gooseberries and blackberries so that my mother could make jam. We'd sit lazily in the sun, chatting about what we'd get up to next. One day I told the lads about Michael – about what a great piano player he was.

'He couldn't play the piano!' one said. 'Sure he can't even serve in the shop. He's always dopey and fast asleep.'

In the lad's opinion Michael was just a dopey old man who dressed weirdly and frightened children.

'He does! He does play the piano,' I argued.

'Have you ever *seen* him play?' another challenged.

'No, not exactly. But I've heard him play.'

'Ah, that's his *radio* playing – you twit! He couldn't play a piano.'

'I'll *prove* it. I'll prove it.' I retorted. 'You wait and see!'

The banter went on and on. Later, when the lads passed by his shop they shouted awful names at him through the door. But I always felt loyal to Michael, as to me he was someone who was special.

Midsummer and the local women baked cakes and collected donations of lemonade, sweets and balloons from the nearby shops. The whole street was having a party, celebrating the opening of the new community hall. The women hung festive decorations along the walls of the hall and a grand piano sat on stage surrounded by thick red velvet curtains. It was a beautiful sunny day outside and the organisers got up on stage to thank all those for coming. Some of the lads heckled, 'Boring, boring.'

Suddenly the two main doors burst open and in walked my father – arm-in-arm with the bold Michael. I couldn't believe it. He was dressed in red velvet coat tails and matching dicky bow – a great big smile across his powdered face.

Everyone stood to cheer and applaud. It was the first time anyone had seen him outside his little shop. My father gave me a wink as he led Michael by the arm on stage, grabbed the microphone and announced to everyone, 'We have our very own gifted pianist with us today – he's going to play some classical music for us all. So I'd like you now to put your hands together and give Michael a very warm welcome.'

Michael bowed shyly as the place erupted, everyone clapping with anticipation.

I looked around the room and saw the lads' mouths drop open. Michael flicked his coat tails behind him and, like a true professional, he sat on the red velvet piano stool and ran his long fingers softly over the keys.

The same heavenly music that I'd heard so often poured from this small, frail man. The atmosphere was electric and as Michael played one piece after another, I glanced around the hall to see everyone sitting completely still. They were spellbound; completely unaware that this prodigy had been living on their doorstep. Each time Michael finished playing they gave him a standing ovation.

My father was congratulated by everyone on getting *'the genius'* out of his shop.

'Willie, did you know Michael could play the piano?' one woman asked. My father smiled politely, looked up at Michael and said, 'He's an angel, isn't he?' as the applause grew louder and louder.

Michael loved the response he got that day. Everyone warmed to him and he quickly became a hero in the community. They asked him to play at children's parties, weddings and other functions.

At Christmas they brought him presents, and invited him home for Christmas dinner. The lads on the road couldn't do enough for him. Each year the locals painted his little shop in bright, vibrant colours. Michael's story was to be an inspiration; it encouraged me to follow my own path, to express my gift – to live my dream.

In the summer months, my mother would sit me in the garden to get the sun on my back and chest. I'd sit for hours in the glowing sunshine, drinking a glass of her home-made lemonade. This helped build my health for the winter months, yet I still had long and frequent absences from school.

Mrs Johnston, the school inspector, was a big woman with a frightening voice. She wore a fox fur, the head and eyes draped over her shoulders, gaping out. Her job was to ensure that all children of school-going age were attending school. I knew her heavy knock on the hall door.

She'd burst in, armed with her thick notebook, detailing my absenteeism to my parents. 'Where is he – where is he?' she'd roar, threatening my parents with court.

'He won't learn anything at home in bed all day,' she'd snap. 'When is he going back to school?'

'When he's good and ready, and not a day before!' my father would roar back. 'Now off with you – and don't ever darken this door again!'

Come hail, rain or snow, she'd always come back – pulling me out of bed, waving her diary in the air and listing off the days I'd missed in school.

My father was very protective of me then. A special bond grew between us.

He was a tall man with golden red hair. Sometimes he grew a beard in the cold winter months. He loved to hill walk, cycle and had a great thirst for knowledge. As manager of Browne and Nolans, the book and stationery company, he knew lots of people and I would often find myself in a judge's chambers listening to my father arguing history with a learned judge and his colleagues.

On his time off, he enjoyed working as a landscape gardener, and when I was well enough, he'd take me with him on the crossbar of his bike. I loved to watch him transform an overgrown garden into a vibrant one, invigorated by his hands into a new period of growth. He stayed close to nature and grew vegetables in the back garden, which kept us supplied all year round.

Understanding that I was at times frail and weak, he kept his pace to mine, never forcing me to do anything that might cause me difficulty or stress. It was a great time of getting to know him better. His interest in me strengthened my resolve to get well.

My mother worked in the local college, dividing her time

between work and looking after me at home.

'His chest isn't great, is it?' Dr Byrne would ask, his cold stethoscope pressed against my thin ribs. We were on another visit to the local health centre.

'His ears are all inflamed. Is he still stammering?'

'Yes, doctor. Some days worse than others.'

'How long is he out of school?'

'It's about a month now, doctor.'

'Well, I'll give him another tonic to keep him going for a few days. But he'll have to go back to school soon. He can't be out all this time, or they'll put him away.'

Red, yellow, orange, pink tonics – they all tasted the same, syrupy and sweet. Sometimes they made me more sick than the illness itself. Granny Brien's medicine was a sip of her mulled stout as we sat by the fire at night, or some wild nettle soup. But I was stuck with these dreadful tonics, which tasted foul and did little to help me; my health was beginning to fail.

Each night I'd wake gasping, wheezing and coughing, a heavy weight pressing down on my chest.

The sound of me gasping for air would wake my brother Billy, who'd remind me *he* had to go to school the next morning.

Sometimes in the middle of the night, I'd steal away to the back garden to breathe in the crisp night air – trying to distract myself with the dogs from the terrible panic I was feeling.

It was two o'clock in the morning. I'd fallen out of bed and woke to find myself on the cold stone floor. My chest was severely congested – it was impossible to breathe.

Panic engulfed me when I reached the back door. I struggled with the two bolts, unsure if I had the strength to open them. The noise woke up the dogs, which sniffed outside the door with quiet excitement. I managed to free the bolts and fell into the crisp night air. The dogs instinctively knew I was in trouble and cowed down to lick my feet.

I collapsed on a sack of turf, and called out, 'Granny Brien, please help me!'

But there was only the sound of the wind, and the drip-drip from the tap on the wall.

My mouth was parched. I struggled to get up on my feet and mustered the last bit of strength I had to reach the tap. As I sipped in the cold water my breathing grew heavier; everything began to spin. I keeled over and started to get sick.

As I lay on the ground, moving in and out of consciousness, my life flashed before me. I called out in the night for help, but there was no one there, only the dogs.

How much more can I take of this, I cried. What was my life all about? I felt alone and in complete despair. I shouted out in anger for God to help me. I could feel my head throbbing, becoming heavier.

Suddenly, out of nowhere, there was a gush of wind and I felt a strong 'presence' envelop me.

I looked up slowly, half afraid as a glowing presence hovered in the air, reaching out to touch me.

The pressure on my chest began to ease. The heavy burden I was carrying melted away. My mind became crystal clear.

Then this presence spoke, 'Everything will be all right. We are here with you. We are with you always. You have come to do important work.'

Immediately I had a vision, as if I had moved forwards in time. I could see myself in a large hall with hundreds of people, my hands on their heads, healing them.

'This is your life's work. Everything will be all right. We will be with you all the time,' the voice spoke again.

It seemed an age before this presence left. Slowly I became aware of the dogs sitting beside me; the noise of the tap dripping; the stars twinkling in the night sky; the hushed sound of the wind as it swept around the corner of the house.

I felt so much better, I wanted to jump up and dance around the garden with excitement, yet I wondered who had spoken to me.

I glanced around the corner of the house – the lilac tree was gently swaying in the wind. I looked in the garden shed but there was nobody there. All the fear I'd been carrying for such a long time had gone; in its place there was a beautiful peace, one that I had never felt before. Suddenly I began to feel the cold, and realised I was standing in the garden in my bare feet, with hardly a stitch on. The dogs wagged their tails, brushing up against me.

'Did you see it, did you see what happened?' I asked. But their excitement grew, as they chased each other around the garden.

I returned to the house, tiptoeing softly through my parents' bedroom, waking my mother who promptly told me to get back to bed and not to wake the whole house.

I sat up in the bed marvelling at what had happened, recalling every detail, very word. Looking out the window at the stars, I asked, 'How can I sleep with such excitement? Who can I tell?'

Billy was fast asleep in his bed, so I decided against waking him. He wouldn't believe me anyway. I wondered about Michael and his gift of music – did the same thing happen to him?

I never forgot my experience that night. It was imprinted on my mind for ever. It became my secret – one I could never share with anyone.

I soon settled back into school, taking each day as it came, the threat of Mrs Johnson, the school inspector, still hanging over me. The teachers were as intent as ever on drumming 'the learning' into us. One used a springy bamboo cane, that wrapped around the hand for double measure. Another used the leg of an oak chair, which was short and swift.

The headmaster used a long blue wooden rod from a child's cot, with a steel bar going through the centre. Six of the best were administered several times a day for one reason or another. I felt sorry for some of the lads, and they for me, when one of us was at the end of a cane.

Many who couldn't do their homework were beaten for their lack of enthusiasm. Others couldn't keep up with the subjects and lagged behind. So I decided to take action and help them out. It's what Granny Brien would have done, I told myself.

That afternoon I arrived home laden with school bags, telling my mother I wanted the peace and quiet of the garden shed to do my homework. She of course was delighted and told my father that I had finally settled into school. My 'homework' continued in this fashion, until one day my mother called me in for tea. I was so absorbed that I didn't hear her footsteps until she pulled open the shed door and found me knee deep in copybooks. She demanded to know who owned all the school bags.

I quickly made some excuse – I was minding them for the lads while they were out playing football.

Mr McManus, the schoolteacher, was extremely happy with his new class of bright and clever pupils. His tough measures, as he put it, were at last paying off.

I was only too delighted that the daily beatings had stopped. Until one morning – while correcting the homework, Mc Manus blew a fuse when he discovered the same mistake in all the copybooks. Up he jumped from his desk and, like a prized greyhound, shot down the aisle at high speed.

'Who's the boy that's cheating in my class?' he shouted angrily.

His cane crashed down on Delaney's desk. Everyone jumped with fright.

'Wait till I get the boy that cheated in my class. His life won't be worth living,' he roared, his anger filling the room.

Stephen Murphy was the most nervous boy in class. McManus knew he was easily intimidated. He came from behind and lashed Murphy's desk with the long bamboo cane. Copybooks flew through the air. Young Murphy jumped out of his skin with fright. He was easy prey.

'It's Hogan, Sir! It's Hogan!' he stammered, and burst into tears.

I dug my head down into my copybook. McManus approached and put his big foot on top of my seat with the point of his shoe digging into my side. I was terrified to look up, my heart thumping.

'Tell us, Hogan ... how did you do it? Better still, *why* did you do it?'

My whole body went numb, my mind full of fear with the thoughts of what was going to happen next. McManus drew his face down to mine.

'Look at me, Hogan, when I'm speaking' he roared, his voice blasting my ear. I shook inside; my mouth parched; I couldn't speak.

The lads felt sorry for me as I was hauled up by the back of the neck in front of the class and dealt with. That day, I went home with blood-red ears, purple arms, purple hands and legs – and only one school bag.

Summer came and the harsh world of school was quickly forgotten. I'd find myself on the bus with Billy, travelling to my grandmother's house, to stay with uncle Christy and aunt Sis. Every day was a great adventure. Christy, Billy and I would head off at dawn to the hills, collecting wild mushrooms, hunting for rabbits or fishing. Christy loved the wildlife and could communicate with just about every bird and animal. His bedroom was crammed with decorative cages he made himself – filled with all kinds of coloured birds. We called it his aviary.

We'd arrive back at the house, well after dusk, laden down with all kinds of berries, wild mushrooms and a few salmon or trout for the supper.

After a while, Aunt Sis married Paddy – a tall, handsome man who loved ballroom dancing. They went everywhere on Paddy's motorbike, winning prizes at dancing competitions throughout the country. Now, Uncle Christy, Paddy and Aunt Sis all lived happily together in Granny Brien's house.

As the holidays drew to a close, my mother and father would join us, telling us the news of our friends 'back home'. It always came as a terrible shock to be told that school started the following Monday. Despite my protests and pleadings to stay in Wicklow, my Da always managed to cajole me back to Dublin and school.

At school, the punishments grew worse. Some of the lads were sent away to industrial schools for poor attendance. Others got into trouble with the law.

I had just turned thirteen when the school was burnt to the ground. What would happen next? I wondered.

CHAPTER 3

IT NEVER RAINS, BUT IT POURS

'The old triangle goes jingle jangle, along the banks of the Royal Canal.'
Brendan Behan

'WAKE UP! QUICK, WAKE UP!' a voice whispered from the darkness. I shot bolt upright in bed, and for a moment thought I was back in the nightmare of school.

'I got you a job, son. Just down the lane,' said my father as he gently shook my arm.

'A job! What job?'

'With Frank. How'd you like to work for Frank Thomson?' he asked, while I got dressed.

Frank Thomson was a sheet metal worker and a mender of cars. Anything there was to know about cars – Frank knew it. His garage was down the lane, beside Mr. Brenner, the bin maker.

I turned up at 8.30 and got instructions from a pair of legs sticking out from underneath a Morris Minor.

'Fetch me a half-inch ring spanner!' Frank shouted, and as I raced down the garage to gape at tools, nuts and bolts, it seemed as if I'd been working there for ever.

'Ring spanners have closed heads – open spanners opened heads!' the voice bellowed from under the car.

Frank was a hard man; hard but fair. Not the sort to talk nicely to people, his school of teaching was the one of hard knocks. One day I swear I saw all the ring spanners dancing on their hooks as Frank let out his usual roar.

'You'll learn nothing with the books,' he'd say. 'It's savvy you need. It's here in the real life you'll become street-wise.'

Of course he was right: I was thirteen years of age and had learnt precious little in school to help me face the world. The work was hard but after all I'd been through it gave me strength and stability.

Frank paid me the princely sum of £2 and 10 shillings a week.

Out of my first week's wages, I had to buy a pair of blue dungarees, which cost £5. My mother made up the rest. She was only too happy to see me start my first real job.

For all his toughness and sharp tongue, Frank was kind to everyone in the community who needed help.

If he wasn't chasing a debtor down the lane with his lump hammer, then he would drop everything to weld a wheel on a pram for a mother who couldn't afford a new one.

I'd been working in Frank's garage for over a year, when a chain of events occurred that would change my life for ever. Monday morning I got up for work, as usual, but sensed a change in the atmosphere at home. My parents seemed ill at ease. My father ate little at breakfast, but just stared at his plate. Billy glanced nervously at my mother. Finally, my father broke the news: a new landlord had purchased both our house and next door, he said, and wanted us out.

'It never rains, but it pours,' my father joked, but there were tears in his eyes.

My heart sank to see my parents in such a terrible state. Many fond memories lay in the house for them; my father's parents had lived there all their lives – my mother moving in from Wicklow when they got married. They knew of nowhere else.

I stepped outside to gather my thoughts. My mind flashed back to Granny Brien, to an afternoon when a woman burst through the door, crying, 'The police are throwin' us on to the street!'

As my grandmother and I caught up with her, we could hear children screaming inside her house. A police sergeant shouted through the letter-box, 'You'll have to leave now. Open this door!'

Granny Brien ran up the garden path, her black shawl blowing in the wind.

'Leave that poor family alone!' she roared, and the sergeant looked around, terrified. 'You hear me?'

'I'm … I'm serving an eviction order, Ma'am. Non-payment of rent,' he stammered. Granny Brien grabbed his bike, plucked him by the neck and threw him on to the street. The gathering crowd laughed and clapped. Granny Brien lifted her shawl – took some coins from her purse – and tossed them at the sergeant's feet.

'There! That will pay the rent for a while' she said, 'Now, off with you. And don't let me see you troubling that poor family again!'

The sergeant picked up the money, quickly mounted his bike and disappeared down the road.

If only Granny Brien was here now, I thought.

A few weeks passed. Frank came into the garage late one morning and asked if my mother was buying new furniture.

'No … why?' I asked.

'Well, your stuff is out on the road,' he said.

A knot formed in my stomach: I looked up towards the house to see beds, wardrobes, tables and chairs piled high on the street with our dogs running wild.

'We're being evicted, Frank,' I said, swallowing hard.

'Where're you moving to?'

'Nowhere, Frank. We've nowhere to go,' I whispered.

I refrained from telling him about our new landlord for fear he might run after him with his lump hammer.

That afternoon my father came looking for me to help out.

'Ah, Willie. I'm sorry to hear about your troubles,' said Frank sympathetically when my father told him the whole story. 'Can no one help?'

'No ... Frank. No,' my father choked.

We managed to move the rest of the furniture before four o' clock, then sat on the street with nowhere to go. My father sat in his favourite armchair on the footpath.

'It's a great view from here – looking down the lane,' he declared, his old Dublin wit shining through. I felt embarrassed as our neighbours passed. Every now and then Frank would shout up from the garage, 'Did you get anywhere, yet, Willie?'

'No, we're still waiting,' my father bantered. 'It's like waiting for a bloody execution!'

Five bells rang out from the town hall clock. My father looked up and rallied with a bar of Brendan Behan's song: 'The old triangle goes jingle jangle, along the banks of the Royal Canal.'

I went into the house for the last time, and opened the back door into the garden.

I recalled the night I was helped by the 'presence' as I lay on the ground, half unconscious, hardly breathing. I looked up once again at the evening sky, closed my eyes and begged the presence for help. A few minutes passed. Distantly, I heard the sound of a car coming up the lane, then pulling up outside. It was a man from the local council. He had the key to a vacant house three miles away, he said. I looked at my parents but they refused to budge. They were determined to stay for ever on the footpath.

I jumped on my bike and cycled off to see this house; key in hand – pedalling as fast as I could.

Broken glass lay everywhere; the windows and doors were boarded up with sheets of galvanised iron. It would take Frank's kango hammer to get us through the door, I thought. But an inner voice kept telling me that things would be all right. Instinctively, I knew that this was to be our new home.

I raced back and told my parents how 'lovely' the new house was – that we should move in immediately.

But they just sat there, reluctant to go, even though it was now cold and dark on the street.

The street light flickered on. We gazed at the face of the town hall clock for the last time; the same clock that had told us the time throughout the years. Alas, time had run out on us now.

'Frank sent me! Do you want your furniture brought some- where?' asked a young man from a blue Volkswagen van. And as my parents looked at one another, I shouted, 'Yes! … Yes we do!' and Billy and I quickly loaded up what we could and headed off.

'Jesus … it's a dive!' exclaimed Billy when he saw our new abode. 'I thought you said it was a lovely house? How do we get in?'

Luckily, the driver had a crow bar and prised the galvanised sheeting off to expose what was left of the hall door. We carried in the furniture and left it sitting on broken glass in the front room.

'Wait till Da and Ma see this place. You'll be murdered!' Billy warned.

My parents stayed at the old house until all the furniture was cleared from the street. Finally, they locked up the family home and moved into our new house under cover of darkness. Thankfully, they hadn't seen the state of the house in daylight. That night we slept soundly on bare floorboards, dead with exhaustion, as the wind outside rattled the house.

Dislocated – as if in a dream, I cycled to work the next morn- ing; weaving through streets and lane-ways, trying to find my bear- ings. Passing our old house on the way – I wondered what had happened to us all.

There was no gas or electricity in our new home. My mother coped by boiling water and cooking over the open fire. We slept on mattresses on the floor – the fire built up during the night for heat. As the wind whistled through cracks in the galvanised tin, our candles threw eerie shadows along the walls.

As I cycled home from work a few nights later, I was surprised to see my father in the old house, sitting alone by the open fire; the rooms laid bare. From then on I'd find him sitting there, alone with all his childhood memories, unable to let go.

We had only been in our new house a couple of weeks, when Uncle Christy arrived at our doorstep. Nervously kneading his cap in hand, he told us how he'd come from Wicklow with bad news. Uncle Paddy was in hospital, he said. He'd been in a bad motorcycle accident; he was in a coma, had lost his leg and was paralysed. The doctors held out little hope of him surviving. Christy looked aghast at the state of the house as my mother made him tea. The bad news seemed to be piling up.

Two days passed. My mother had gone to work early. Billy and myself were fast asleep on the floor, when a loud banging on the galvanised window startled us. I peered through a hole to see a squad car outside.

'Paddy must have died,' said Billy as he pulled open the makeshift door.

'Is your mother here?' a policeman asked suspiciously.

'No … she's gone to work.'

'Which one of you is the eldest?'

'I am,' Billy mumbled.

'Can you come with us to the hospital? the policeman asked coldly.

'What for?'

'We need you to identify a body,' the policeman snapped.

Billy looked back at me apprehensively as they sped him away in the squad car.

Later, he identified the body. It was our Da. He had been found dead in the old house the previous night, and brought to the hospital for a post-mortem.

My heart sank; the nightmare wasn't over – it was getting worse. A dark cloud had descended, but there was no time to take it all in.

After my father's funeral, another knock came to the hall door. It was a neighbour with a telephone message: 'Uncle Christy was dying in hospital. Could we come quick?'

We dropped everything and caught the bus to Granny Brien's house in Wicklow, still assuming that the neighbour had got the information mixed up; surely she meant Uncle Paddy was dying and not Christy? The news was confirmed, however. Uncle Christy had just died from a brain haemorrhage – but it was in the Richmond hospital back in Dublin and not in Wicklow. We were in the wrong place and devastated by the news. It seemed that everything we had was now lost.

I decided to stay on in Wicklow. Aunt Sis had her hands full; making the funeral arrangements for Uncle Christy, and running into the hospital to see her husband, Paddy. She needed my help.

Paddy made a slow recovery and eventually came home, a far cry from the man he once was. To make ends meet, Aunt Sis went back to work. Paddy's leg had been amputated below the hip, and had failed to heal. His right arm was still paralysed. No longer able to work, he became despondent and depressed.

But time heals all wounds and, while Uncle Paddy's wounds were visible, mine were deep inside; I felt we were all going through a major healing of some kind.

Months passed in a fog. Summer was approaching and gradually the shock eased. Aunt Sis broached the subject of a job for me in Christy's old place – the coffin-making factory where he had worked all his life.

The next morning I stood at Christy's work bench; all his tools still neatly arranged there, and I felt a strange shiver creep over me.

'You don't look like your uncle,' the forty-odd workers teased.

'Dublin jackeens – ye think yer tough!' younger fellas taunted and challenged me to a fight. Late in the evening, they'd send me in to the morgue to fetch a 'glass hammer' or a 'round square' – close the door and turn the lights out. I had my work cut out if I was to survive this new environment, I reckoned.

Eventually, with an odd bruise here and there, I earned their respect and was favourably known as 'the worker'.

I learned everything about coffin making; about American oak, prana pine from Brazil, beech from Africa, elm from Canada. Every month I was sent to the docks to select the best wood that came in great big ships from all over the world.

We made children's and babies' coffins, paupers' coffins. Caskets with high domed lids; hand-polished, waxed, lacquered, pitched and leaded, with fabric beadings and coloured linings. I put in headstones and dug many a grave across Wicklow.

We had four big old hearses, and a number of limousines. Alfie, one of the old hearse drivers, would take me to Dublin airport, to collect the remains that came from far away exotic places; Egypt, Australia, America or Africa.

Sometimes, we'd collect an urn filled with ashes, a file about the person's life attached. It made fascinating reading, as we skipped back home over the mountains into Wicklow.

The news was rife that Eamon de Valera, the President of Ireland, was on the point of dying. I remembered the time 'Old Dev' – as my father called him, took the Easter salute outside the GPO in O'Connell Street, while the Irish army marched proudly past. Little did I realise that one day I'd be helping to make up his casket.

I was back in Granny Brien's world and soon began to settle into my new life. When I wasn't looking after Paddy on lunch breaks, or in the evenings after work, I'd go for long walks, read books or go to the cinema where Granny Brien sneaked me in under her black shawl as a child.

The films of Bruce Lee – the kung fu expert – appealed to me. I became interested in his philosophy and read everything about him. A karate class started in the local community hall. I joined, and trained under Professor Suzuki (Seventh Dan) and five martial artists.

Learning to speak some Japanese, I worked my way up to brown belt, the grade before black, and gave my first karate class.

I became interested in the 'katas' – a series of concentrated movements that demanded skill, focus and discipline. I studied t'ai chi, an ancient Chinese philosophy of movement, which allows the 'chi', the universal energy, to flow through the mind and body. My introduction to yoga, however, brought the wardrobe crashing down, breaking the mirror, as I attempted my first head stand.

Meditation helped me tune into the invisible world – the world of spirit. I received messages intuitively and wrote them in a journal that I kept on my bedside table.

Karate, t'ai chi and yoga gave me a strength I never had before. Before going to sleep at night, I'd meditate on the purpose of my life. 'Surely there was more to my life than working in the undertakers?' I reasoned, in the darkness.

One chilly November night, I went out for my usual run after work. There wasn't a soul about. It was a night for sitting by the fire. I'd been running for twenty minutes, along a country road overgrown with trees and ivy, when suddenly I was startled by a voice that rooted me to the ground.

'This part of your life is over,' the voice boomed. 'This part of your life is over.' I looked around and saw three angel-like figures, hovering above me.

My mind started to spin and then expand. I felt I was leaving my body.

'We are with you, and have been with you. All through your life.'

'Who are you, what do you want?' I asked.

'We have been with you since you were born,' a gentle voice echoed.

Suddenly I remembered my birth – coming out of the caul into the world.

My life flashed before me. I saw myself in a large hall, healing people, just like I'd seen before.

Another flash and I saw myself in the undertakers, being handed a piece of paper by my boss. Then walking in the rain, up a narrow road into a small office, drying my hair with a towel next to a plump man with red, matted hair.

I felt myself returning to my body. The three angel-like figures still hovered around me.

'It was you who came to my rescue, when I was a child in the garden,' I cried.

The gentle voice spoke again. 'We will be with you and guiding you all the time.'

Then there was a silence as my mind filled up with questions. The voice continued. 'Call, we will be there. Go with the changes.'

As they left, I suddenly became aware of the cold night air. A strange excitement rushed through me. I remembered what happened when I was a child in the garden – I remembered being healed. I punched the night air and shouted, 'It was real! It did happen. It's happened again!' I cried. 'It's happened again …!'

As the experience began to wear off, I became aware of the path I'd been running on; the branches of the trees above moving; the wall full of ivy. I jumped up on the wall and looked about. All was quiet. I walked up and down the road several times, going over and over in my mind what had happened, remembering every word, retracing every step.

Aunt Sis and Paddy were laughing at a Morecambe and Wise programme on the television when I came through the door.

'He looks like he's seen a ghost,' I overheard Sis whisper as I said my goodnights and climbed the stairs. That night, I wrote it all down in my journal and fell into a deep sleep.

'Quick, quick, get up! Wake up, wake up, wake up!' Sis shouted as she burst into my room. 'Your job is on fire! They need help to put the fire out!'

The room was in complete darkness. It was three o'clock in the morning. I fell back on my pillow thinking I must be dreaming – words thundering through my mind, 'This part of your life is now over. This part of your life is …'. I shot out of bed, got dressed and ran downstairs.

As I turned the street corner I could see the undertakers engulfed in flames. A plume of smoke and fire shot from the rooftops. Support beams buckled and fell with a hail of sparks to the ground. Firemen doused the flames. My workmates and I ran with buckets of water, back and forth to the inferno, until dawn broke on the horizon.

The following days passed in a dream. We cleaned up the mess as best we could and painted a wall or two. It was a very insecure time for us all, especially the older men. I was happy I had a job – even if it consisted of a burnt-out shell. But it was not to be. Early one morning I was called into the office and bluntly told I was being let go. As the boss handed me a reference, my mind flashed back to the encounter on the road that night. Was this all meant to be? I wondered.

The school fire and the undertakers had closed chapters in my life. What was going to happen next? Putting a few things in my pocket, I boarded the bus for Dublin, just like I'd done when Granny Brien passed away. I was seventeen years of age.

Those years in Wicklow had passed swiftly. Now I was back in my mother's house – dislocated, suffering from shock and trauma. It all began tumbling in on me. I hit rock bottom.

The rain pelted from the heavens on a bleak December morning.

I put on my leather jacket and walked the empty streets to help ease my inner pain. Sheets of icy rain formed gullies in the streets, soaking me to the skin.

In a trance, I veered off the main road and up a narrow laneway. Something told me I'd been here before. An open door led into a small office building. I found myself in a long passageway, looking into three small offices. A tall, plump man, in his forties, with red hair, saw me through the glass.

'Are you here for the job?' he asked in a soft Yorkshire accent.

'Yes', tumbled out before I had time to think.

'Did you see the ad in the newspapers?'

'No,' I whispered, and felt the pain of having no job.

'You look a sorrowful sight, laddie. Sit here in the warm office,' he beckoned and returned moments later with a large white towel.

'Here, dry yourself with that.'

As I began drying my hair, I suddenly realised, that this office, this man, the white towel was all part of the vision I had while out running that night in Wicklow.

'You're a little late,' he continued. 'I've already interviewed over a hundred applicants in the last week alone.'

He looked at me with a kindly smile, introduced himself as Malcolm, and acted as if we'd known each other all our lives. The office door swung open and in walked a cheerful middle-aged woman with tea and biscuits.

'Where did you work before?' Malcolm enquired.

Initially I was fearful of telling him about the undertakers. But an inner voice told me to trust him.

As the wind and rain howled outside, I told Malcolm about my time in Wicklow; about the dreadful fire that had destroyed everything.

'You know, I've a strange feeling about you,' he said smiling. 'I think you would be the perfect man for the job.'

My heart skipped a beat when he said, 'I know it may sound strange, but I feel you've been sent here.'

How did he know who sent me? I wondered. Was he an angel in human form?

'Can you start in the morning?'

'Yes – Yes!' I blurted out, and hope lit up inside me.

I was waking up, very slowly, from this dreadful nightmare. I had found myself, not a stone's throw from my house, working in Malcolm's electrical engineering company.

At last I had a job, an identity. Yet, I'd seen the invisible world and wanted to know more. I devoted all my spare time now to meditation, communicating with my 'invisible friends' from the spirit world.

To heighten my awareness, I fasted on distilled water. I tried apple, grape and pear fasts; any fruit I could lay my hands on.

The first Irish health food shop opened in Trinity Street, in Dublin in the mid 1960s. It stocked a small selection of vitamins and minerals. But for me it was like a magnet; I felt completely at home there.

I researched diet, herbs and vitamins, noting the effects they had on my mind and body. Practising breathing exercises in front of a mirror, I'd notice the colours around me brighten, change and expand. The same coloured light pulsated from my fingertips.

I studied the energies that surrounded people. I noticed that when they were downbeat or sad, the glow around them was dimmer. When they were upbeat and happy, the glow was brighter.

In my spare time, I was drawn to the National Art Gallery. There I would sit for hours, gazing at the religious icon paintings; not knowing why I was there, until one day, I realised I was drawn not just to the figures in the paintings, but also to what surrounded the heads of these figures – the halo.

The halo and the colours I saw around people were one and the same. It was the spirit of the person I was seeing. From that moment on a veil lifted – the invisible world became visible.

My workmates, however, talked of summer holidays, buying a car and finishing their apprenticeship. I was straddling two worlds, feeling isolated and alone.

'What are you looking at?' a lad asked suspiciously when he caught me looking over his head. The rest always stared agog when I produced home-made brown bread and apple juice for lunch. They thought I'd just come down in a spaceship.

Outside work however, I was gradually getting a reputation as someone who knew how to transform people's health through diet and vitamins. I took up hatha yoga – this time learning how to do a head stand properly. I was introduced to like-minded people and immediately felt at home in their company.

In the health shop one day, I was looking at a bottle of vitamin E capsules, selling at the pricely sum of £13.99, when a slim booklet fell from the shelf. The word 'auras' shot out at me like a thunderbolt. I opened its pages, and my heart quickened when I read the following:

> *'Ever since I can remember, I have seen colours in connection with people. I do not remember a time when the human beings I encountered did not register on my retina with blues and greens and reds gently pouring from their heads and shoulders. It was a long time before I realised that other people did not see these colours; it was a long time before I heard the word aura, and learned to apply it to this phenomenon which to me was commonplace. I do not ever think of people except in connection with their auras; I see them change in my friends and loved ones as time goes by. Sickness, dejection, love, fulfilment, these are all reflected in the aura and for me the aura is the weathervane of the soul. It shows which way the winds of destiny are blowing.'*

The booklet was about a man who could see auras throughout his life. His name was Edgar Cayce. He lived from 1877 to 1945, near Hopkinsville, Kentucky in the United States.

Known as 'the Sleeping Prophet', Edgar Cayce spent the best

part of his life in a trance-like state, giving psychic readings, information on diet, vitamins, herbs and on the deeper spiritual aspects of life.

The more I read about the man, the more affinity I felt towards him.

At the age of six, he too had a vision, which told of his future; of the extraordinary work he would be doing when he grew older. It was no accident that our paths had crossed.

A few years later I would meet the woman who had compiled the booklet that fell from the shelf that day. Her name was Elsie Sechrist and she had been Edgar Cayce's secretary for many years. Elsie was in the Hibernian Hotel in Dublin, reading and interpreting auras. Knowing something of my abilities, she asked me to share the platform with her. This gave me more confidence to develop my gift further.

I spent many hours looking at people's auras, as they passed me on the street. Some had unusual colours; all different shapes and sizes. I soon began to identify what each colour meant.

Inevitably, the time came when I began to lose interest in my job. Too much had happened to me over the years; I'd had experiences I just couldn't ignore. I realised it was time to take responsibility; to somehow express the divine gift I'd been born with.

When I handed in my notice, Malcolm took it badly.

'Is it more money you want?' he asked.

'You've been very kind and understanding,' I assured him.

'Is it promotion you're after – family problems?'

Poor Malcolm tried his best to keep me there; but how could I tell him about my new life – where would I start? Eventually, we parted on good terms, and my life as a healer began.

My very first healing experience happened late one evening after a lecture. I'd returned with a group of like-minded people to a house for tea. As we sat around the fire chatting, our host asked us to keep the noise level down. Her mother was in the next room, she said, suffering with a severe migraine headache.

'Ask your mother does she want healing?' one of the group prompted. 'Tell her there's a man here with us tonight who might help her.' To my surprise, the girl returned a few minutes later and asked me to follow her.

'If you could help Mammy, I'd be most delighted,' she said anxiously, opened a door and told me to go in.

Inside, the curtains were drawn and a dim light glowed in the corner. I introduced myself to the poor woman who was curled up in agony on the sofa.

There were black rings under her eyes and pain etched itself across her sunken face. She looked up at me in a daze and quietly whispered, 'I've had this awful migraine for over three weeks now. If you could do something to ease it, I'd be truly grateful.'

'I'll try my best,' I assured her and placed my hands gently on her throbbing head. Immediately, I felt a surge of healing power flow through my hands, then through the muscles of her head, neck and shoulder blades. Beneath my hands I could feel intense energy penetrate her frail body, dispersing all the pain away.

The response was instant; the woman let out a deep sigh of relief. Finally, when the healing power stopped flowing, I opened my eyes and took my hands away.

Looking over the woman's head, I could see the light around her expanding. It was glowing now with a new radiance. She lay still for a while in that peaceful state as I left the room. Ten minutes later she was in the front room, entertaining her guests.

'You know, when my daughter told me there was a man who could heal in the house, I said it would take a bloody miracle to lift this whopper of a headache,' she laughed as she told everyone of her healing experience.

At our weekly group meetings we would practise a number of exercises. In order to heighten our psychic abilities we would sit quietly with eyes closed, and focus our attention on the centre of the forehead, which we referred to as the third eye, or the psychic gland. With practice, some would feel a pulsating sensation, in and around the forehead – a clear indication that the doors to our psychic abilities were opening. Sometimes we received helpful information from the psychic world, which we'd share in the group.

This information sometimes came as an impression, or a clear voice; advising and giving us a purpose to our lives.

My own psychic abilities became more frequent. I communicated daily with my invisible friends, and was taught by the finest spirit minds. Up to then I could see only the outline of the aura. With practice, I began to see each aura separately – where it originated from – and where it was blocked. I realised that the aura was functioning through the seven major glands of the body. I also learnt about the chakra system – the wheels that propel energy through the body.*

When my psychic sensitivity became more heightened I would glimpse my invisible friends, in spirit form, moving around the room. Eventually, I was able to see them in almost human form.

When word got out that I had healed the woman of migraine, a steady trickle of people came. A kind friend, Moira, lent me a room, and I began to heal in earnest.

Tom, a recent member of our group, was very interested in spiritual and psychic matters. I had arranged to meet him one weekend, to talk further about the whole realm of the spirit world. During that week, I had promised Moira that I would paint a number of bedrooms upstairs in her house, to repay her kindness. By Thursday I'd made good headway, and finished painting the walls and ceiling in the last room. I glanced at my watch; it was coming up to five o'clock. The bedroom door was open. I put down the paintbrush

---

* I describe the chakra system and auras in more detail in Chapter 5.

on the rim of the paint can, then checked my pockets to see whether I had enough money for an evening newspaper. Suddenly, I felt a presence behind me.

I went to turn around – thinking someone had just come in – but remembered that no one would be home until after six. Yet the presence was so overpowering.

I quickly turned around to see a man standing by the bedroom door.

With a jolt it took me a moment to realise that it was Tom from our little group, staring anxiously at me from across the room.

'Hello, Tom,' I said nervously. 'How did you know I was here?'

'I've gone over, Tony. I've gone over,' he said urgently.

As if in a dream, I heard myself say, 'I'll see you on Saturday in town as arranged.' How did Tom get into the house? I wondered. The front door was locked. I remembered checking it earlier.

'Tony, I've gone over. I've been drowned in the sea. I've gone over. You're the only one who understands. I've tried telling my sister, Betty, and my family. But they don't realise,' he said, as his presence shimmered and faded in and out.

'Will you tell them I'm all right? he asked fretfully. 'I didn't feel a thing ...'

'It's all right, Tom. I understand. I'll deliver the message. Go on. Go to where you have to. Everything will be all right here,' I said.

The words seemed to flow from my tongue – a distant echo of what I once heard before. Tom smiled one last time, then vanished into a silvery blue mist.

I made sure the key of the house was still in my pocket, checked the hall door and, in a dream, walked around to Paddy, the paper man, on the street corner.

The soft evening sun was still shining. The rush hour traffic building up. Paddy turned to me and said 'Look what they did to me eye, the bastards!'

'What happened?' I asked as normally as I could.

'I've been down to that cursed place, the Eye n'Ear Hospital, this morning,' he said angrily. 'They put a great big needle into me eye, and nearly blinded me, the savages.'

Part of me was still in the conversation with Tom – 'I've gone over, Tony,' – while the other was on the street with Paddy.

As Paddy kept up his banter, I noticed a headline on his billboard: 'Man Missing – Feared Drowned'. Paddy handed me an *Evening Herald* from under his arm with a picture of Tom and the headline 'Man Feared Drowned While Swimming In Sea', across the front page.

Cars beeped on the busy street corner. Paddy zig-zagged through them with his newspapers.

I walked slowly back to the house, reading the headline; my hands shaking as I remembered Tom's words, like vapour running through my mind. 'I've gone over, Tony. I've gone over.'

I had begun to give public lectures on diet and auras, teaching people how to use their minds to self-heal. A young businessman, named Paul, wanted to know all about healing and spiritual philosophy. I had healed him once of psoriasis – an 'incurable' skin condition. Now Paul wanted to bring healing to others. He would set up clinics across the country, he said, and drive me there.

'There's lots of people Tony, who badly need your help,' he insisted.

Eventually I agreed: I would see people two mornings a week in Dublin, and travel the country mid-week with Paul. We'd set off early in the evenings, before the traffic had time to build up, and drive to hotels, houses and parish halls.

People were in dreadful pain from chronic arthritis, a slipped disc or shingles. Many had cancer. Depression, nervous breakdowns, panic attacks and alcoholism were common. Everywhere we went we found suicide and despair.

'Are you the bone-setter?' they'd ask when we showed up. 'Do you have the cure – any good at getting rid of ringworm?' an old man asked. Most of them couldn't afford to stay in hospital or pay for medical care.

'Had ye been here a week ago, ye may have been able to help poor Tom Rice. Suffered all his life with bad depression,' an old woman told me. 'He committed suicide, the poor soul.'

Steadily my confidence grew – I was receiving hundreds of letters from grateful patients.

Daily, I witnessed the lifting of depression; the flexibility returning to a woman's arthritic back as she tipped her toes. An old woman's weeping leg ulcer dried up and healed before my very eyes.

Travelling the lonely country roads with Paul, my mind would drift back to Granny Brien. I could see her sitting by her cosy log fire, knitting needles in hand.

'You are a special child', she had told me then. And, as I looked out the car window at the passing fields, I realised that healing was my gift.

Word travels fast in the country; each week there were crowds of new faces; new diseases to heal.

'You cured my neighbour of crippling arthritis, that's why I'm here.'

'Mrs Philips, who works in the local post office, got great relief from your healing powers. She's a new woman.'

'Me uncle, Tom, had painful gout in his legs and feet. Now he's back working on the farm again. You're the man that cured him. He sends his regards and his missus will be along herself in due course.'

It was a great time of learning and meeting new people; going from county to county, from farm to farm; healing those who were at times too sick to get out of bed.

I remember the first visit to Dundalk – hundreds showed up that evening. They all piled into the great ballroom, chatting excitedly. Many had come from all parts of Northern Ireland, from towns and villages along the border.

I put my head around the door, and couldn't help but notice that everyone had plastic or brown paper bags, either on their laps, or on the floor beside them. Each bag seemed heavy and bulging. A hush came over the room as I walked in. Immediately, they hauled their bags on to their laps. I hesitated a moment, trying to gauge the air of anticipation in the room. A woman in the front row caught my eye and spoke in a low northern voice, 'Tony, do you know what you want to do?'

'Yes,' I said, clearing my throat. 'I'll start here and work my way around the room.'

The woman got up from her chair, came up to me and whispered, 'Do you not see? Everyone has brought their clay.'

Thinking I was in some sort of pottery class, I asked, 'What's the clay for?'

'The clay! You don't know what the clay is for? What sort of a healer are you?' she teased.

'Tony will be back in one moment!' she announced and beckoned me out of the hall.

A loud burst of conversation filled the room. Everyone wondered what was up.

I could tell by the woman's manner that she had never met anyone like me before.

'You mean you don't know about the clay?'

I looked puzzled. But like a schoolteacher preaching to a young child, she said, 'All the people with the clay go to the faith healer from the North. You take a pound of clay from a relative's grave on a moonlit night, the legend goes.

All you have to do, Tony, is to put your hands around the bags and bless the clay. There'll be a bloody riot in there if you don't.'

I had visions of people walking the graveyards of Ireland at night, shovels and lamps in hand.

'I don't know what the custom is, where you come from, Tony. But that's the custom here.'

'What do they do with the clay after I bless it?' I asked, nervously.

'We all go home and empty the blessed clay into a basin of water, rub the paste all over and then go to bed.'

'My husband doesn't mind at all,' she laughed. He's got used to it by now.

The next morning you wash it off. Away goes all the badness with it. That's the custom.'

In the mean time, Paul was talking to more people who'd just arrived. Turning anxiously to me he said, 'For God's sake, Tony, are you ready? You better get a move on. We've to be up in Monaghan in an hour.'

I followed the woman back inside and, as I began, she kept smiling over at me. Quickly I tuned in to my invisible friends for advice. It would have to be a compromise, I knew. I would put one hand on the person, the other on the clay and give them both healing.

Weeks later, I told them I would prefer to heal people, and not bags of clay. Many were hugely relieved.

'That's great!' a woman cried, as her friends fell around the place laughing. 'I won't be dirtying the sheets tonight.'

In the small hours of the morning, Paul and I would return exhausted to Dublin, marvelling at the remarkable healings we had witnessed that night, Paul's car laden down with food and flowers and plants. People would pay me with loaves of bread; with apple tarts, eggs, blackberry jam; and with bags of potatoes and vegetables they'd grown themselves.

Before dawn broke over the city. Paul would deliver the flowers and plants to the children's hospital, the excess food to the homeless.

I had little money, but my mother helped me out as best she could. 'Give up that old job, son,' she'd say. 'It's not worth it – it won't pay you.'

Several years of healing slipped by. I had established myself as a spiritual healer around the country villages, but I knew that our travels in the country were coming to an end. I had learned a lot and now I needed to focus on my work in Dublin. Paul's business was also steadily growing, so we finally decided that we would each go our separate ways. It had been a magical few years for both of us.

CHAPTER 4

THE HEALING EXPERIENCE

'Healing is a personal gift, which can belong only to those whose natures are compassionate and who radiate love in themselves, and express it for others in their way of life.'

Harry Edwards

I SOON SETTLED DOWN to my practice in Dublin and began to live with this gift. At times it was a burden. Other times inspirational, even magical. There was much to learn.

Today, I never know what I'm faced with when someone comes through my door. Some come on crutches, in wheelchairs, some minus a limb. Some come coughing, wheezing, shaking, stammering, bandaged up in plaster of Paris, surgical corsets, metal braces, walking frames, titanium bolts, surgical slings, some using tranquillisers, morphine, antidepressants, painkillers, lotions, potions, inhalers, nasal sprays, eye drops and ice packs.

'Rotten bones in me neck, Mr Hogan!' said an elderly lady as I opened the door. I could see the pain etched across her face. The colours in her aura were barely visible.

'Come in,' I said and carefully I linked her arm and sat her on the chair.

A young girl followed, dressed in a dark blue cardigan and nurse's uniform.

'My name is Mrs Kennedy, Mr Hogan. But you can call me Olive. This here is Mary the nurse who works with me doctor. Only for her, I wouldn't be able to come to see you this morning. She's the driver,' she laughed.

'What's the problem?' I enquired.

'It's rotten bones in me neck, Mr Hogan. I've had them fifteen long years. Me doctor, Dr Gallagher, tried his best over the years to stop the pain, but he can't do it any more. So he sent me to you. I'm going out of me mind with the pain. It's at me night and day. Look, I can't move me neck, Mr Hogan. They're all rotten. All the bones is rotten,' she exclaimed.

Mary the nurse nodded her head in agreement, then took up the story.

'Dr Gallagher has sent Olive to four hospitals over the years but all the tests show that the bones in Olive's neck have collapsed and disintegrated. That's why her neck is locked in the one position.'

I could see clearly what she meant; Olive's chin looked as if it was welded to her chest.

'She's on the strongest painkilling injections, Mr Hogan. The tablets no longer work. Now, even the injections don't ease her pain.'

Mary went on to explain that Olive had recently been back and forth to the hospital for more scans on her back and neck. But there was nothing more they could do for her.

'Dr Gallagher heard about you from some of his patients. He's retiring soon. Olive is his oldest patient, and he doesn't want to just leave her the way she is.'

When Mary had finished I turned to Olive and said, 'Dr Gallagher must be a very kind-hearted man, to be so concerned about you.'

Olive smiled and said, 'He's always been good to me over the years. Now that I can't get out, he comes to see me every day at home, to give me the injections.' She paused as she adjusted herself on the chair.

'Please, can you help me Mr Hogan? Please?' She pleaded. 'I can't even put me head on the pillow at night to sleep. The pain. Oh, the pain! I'm going out of me mind with it.' Tears began rolling down her cheeks.

'I'll see what I can do for you, Olive,' I replied, while earnestly asking my spirit friends to intercede.

Mary sat across the room, observing everything, taking in my every move. I stood behind Olive and immediately felt the healing power flowing through my hands, as they began to vibrate. Then, closing my eyes, I placed my hands gently on Olive's neck. Within a few minutes, I could feel all the lifeless muscles in her neck twitching, jumping madly, followed by a number of crunching sounds. I continued to where the healing power needed to go until it stopped.

I snapped back into the room to see Olive swinging her head from side to side.

'Look, Mr Hogan, look. The pain's all gone! The pain's all gone! Look, me neck is free!'

The room filled up with excitement. I took a few steps back, observing what had happened.

'Mr Hogan, I can see your clock on the far wall,' she shouted.

'Now, I can see your calendar on the other wall, Mr Hogan.'

Olive began calling out the names of all the objects on the walls as they caught her eye.

'Look, Mary, I can turn me neck!' she laughed. 'I can turn me head. I can look directly at you Mary. All the pain's gone!'

Olive clapped her hands with the excitement of a young child. I glanced over at Mary – with her mouth wide open.

'I can't believe it!' Mary said. 'Its just amazing. I'd never have believed it – only I've seen it with my own eyes.'

'I wonder, Olive, what Dr Gallagher would think of that?' I asked.

'Wait 'til he sees me Mr Hogan! I don't think he'll believe it.'

Out the door they went; Olive swinging her head from side to side; laughing all the way down the stairs.

When I look back at all of the wonderful healings that have taken place I think of how privileged I am to have been born with such a wonderful gift. Day in and day out I meet those who are sick and incurable; their lives unbearable. They are at their wits' end as to what to do or where to turn. By the time most people have come to see me, they have been everywhere else and none of the conventional treatments have worked. I am usually their last port of call. Most have been through the medical end of things and have had all the tests, assessments, X-rays and scans, and a diagnosis made.

I always encourage patients to continue with their medication and continue seeing their doctors. Spiritual healing is complementary to orthodox medicine and works alongside it.

When patients come through the door for the first time, they find themselves in the waiting room. There they can read some of the testimonies from grateful patients who have already been healed or meet those still coming who can give them a first-hand account of their own healing.

When they enter my healing room, they'll see that I keep it simple. There is a vase of flowers on the desk, a few chairs and a treatment couch. On one of the walls there are various certificates from courses I have taken over the years: psychology, counselling, homeopathy and naturopathy – all an extension of my healing work. One certificate of which I am particularly proud is from the National Federation of Spiritual Healers (NFSH). This is an organisation that registers gifted healers who can offer, over a period of time, authentic evidence of spiritual healing. This I was able to achieve early on in my work and I became the first 'Spiritual Healing' member in Ireland.

The NFSH was first established in Britain in 1953 by Harry

Edwards, Gordon Turner and John Britnell. These were the first group of professional healers to come together under one banner, and consisted of five hundred healers. Their aim was to bring spiritual healing to the public and have it accepted as a therapy by the medical profession. Today there are over seven thousand professional healing members of the NFSH, who all work within a code of conduct and who have recently been recognised by the British Medical Association, the Royal College of Physicians, the Royal College of Surgeons and the Royal College of Nursing.

I begin each day with a few moments of meditation. I close my eyes, and attune myself to God, the source of all healing.

During this process I become aware of a heightened sensitivity within my energy fields. The energy centres open. I can feel them vibrating throughout my body. Then a surge of energy passes down through me, centring in and around my forehead and in the palms of my hands.

With my energy fields open the patient's condition will register within me. If the patient is suffering with a migraine, for example, I will experience the exact same headache. Or an ulcer will show itself as a burning in my stomach. If the patient has depression I will experience the same dark cloud pressing on my mind.

I usually weave all these psychic impressions into the conversation. I might hear myself ask, 'Do you have a headache over your right eye? Is your stomach burning? How long have you suffered with depression?' When I get a positive response I know I'm on the right track.

In their auras I will sometimes see flashes of their past, present and future. My spirit friends will also guide me.

I may be told that the person has been in a car crash or had a recent bereavement. They may feel angry and resentful about a private family matter. There may be tensions in the workplace or guilt over something in the past.

Angela worked as a secretary in the bank. She was suffering with high blood pressure and migraine. As she was about to sit down, I asked, 'Who's bullying you at work?' She was totally flabbergasted.

'How did you know about that?' she asked. 'There's only one other person in the whole world that knows about it. That's my older sister Lisa, who lives in New York.'

Sometimes the impressions I pick up seem to have no bearing on what the person is telling me at the time. But a few weeks later they will return and say, 'Remember what you said to me the last time – well it's happened!'

I am very conscious never to use negative language to anybody who comes to see me, regardless of their problem.

I never say I can't help somebody. Experience has taught me over the years that nothing is impossible. My healing gifts have shown there are only possibilities. The source of all healing comes from God, the creator of life, and I am the channel.

When healing, I always maintain a strong energy field around me. This helps to disperse any negative energies that can flow from the patient. Contact healing is where I make contact with my hands on the place or area where the person is experiencing their illness. The traditional name for this is the 'laying on of hands'. Today it is known as 'hand healing' and for some healers one hand gives out a stronger current than the other. This is commonly known as the power hand. Through developing my gift over time I find I am able to transmit the same volume of power through both hands.

Every healing experience is different for me, even with the same person. Sometimes it's focused like a laser beam, while at other times it expands right out, filling the room.

When I feel my hands vibrate strongly, this tells me there is a tremendous surge of power flowing through me at that particular moment.

The more serious the illness, the stronger the power becomes. When I stand near the person, I can see areas within them that are depleted of energy. These feel like icy cold spots, which dictate where and for how long I will place my hands.

Before I call in the next patient I allow a few minutes for the atmosphere to settle back in my healing room. I can feel quite drained after a healing, especially if the person is depressed or seriously ill. So I need time for myself to boost my own energies.

There are times I may need to clear the room of trauma or negativity that can linger long after the person has left.

I try to have as few people as possible in the room while I am healing. I am especially cautious if there is a member of the family who is sceptical or negative towards the healing. This kind of attitude will quickly irritate and drain me, which can inhibit my ability to give free-flowing energy to the patient.

Sometimes I will play uplifting music to help create the right atmosphere. It allows both myself and the patient to move more easily into a relaxed state for the healing to be absorbed.

Usually I will sit in front of the person and feel guided as to where I need to deliver the healing energies. I may feel the urge to put my hands on someone's back even though they are suffering with a knee problem. This is because the knee problem is originally coming from the back.

The healing power flows down my arms and into my hands. The energy flow is in various qualities and strengths.

My hands will tingle and vibrate, from its power, especially my fingertips and centre palms.

If I open my eyes, I will see streams of coloured light pulsating from my hands. This pulsating light flows into the patient's aura moving to where it needs to go.

I leave my hands on the patient for as long as the healing power flows; it can be minutes or sometimes longer, depending on how much healing is required. This can vary from person to person, from treatment to treatment. When sufficient healing energy is given, I automatically break contact by gently taking my hands away. If I don't break contact at the correct moment, the healing current will run in the opposite direction – back up my arms – giving me an unpleasant electric shock! This used to happen frequently in the early days, until my spirit friends showed me when to break contact.

After a healing, some people experience such a charge of energy that they become more active in themselves and want to talk. Others just sit completely silent and serene for quite some time afterwards; enrobed in a mantle of peace and tranquillity.

When I am healing a number of ailments my hands automatically pick up all the places that require healing. I will scan my hand through the person's energy field, and when I come upon the spot my hand will stick to the area like a magnet and the healing energies will flow to the area.

Whenever a distressed mother comes with a sick baby in her arms, I will put my hands gently on the mother's shoulders and transmit the healing power to her. After a few moments the same healing energy will pass through her into the baby. It's wonderful to watch both of them being healed at the same time – the baby calms down and the mother brightens up.

Each person experiences different sensations during a healing session. Some will burst out laughing, while others will end up crying. Many describe seeing vivid colours in their mind's eye, or the room much brighter than before. A sense of peace and relaxation is the most common experience of all.

There are those who feel healing as a warmth, spreading throughout the body, right down the legs, or a tangible heat sensation in the area of illness. Others describe it as a vibration or tingling – like a mild current of electricity coming from my hands and passing through them. All these experiences are definite indications of the healing treatment working.

At the initial appointment a person's energy levels may be very low. On these occasions, the healing power will need to be so strong that every part of the body seems to shake. Some will experience healing at such a deep level that they can't stand up afterwards. This is because their physical energy body, their aura, has been vibrated so much by the healing power, that they can feel disorientated for a while.

When this happens I will ask them to close their eyes and sit still on the chair for a few minutes, or lie on the treatment couch, while the healing energies are being absorbed into the physical body.

Of course, not everyone feels something, especially at the first visit. The patient may be too stressed-out or too wrapped up with their own problems to notice anything. It can be quite funny, however, to see their reaction after a number of healing sessions – when the problem has subsided and they are more relaxed and balanced within themselves. They can look quite shocked when they feel all the healing sensations flowing into them.

Sadly, however, there are those who are closed to my healing; they say they don't feel anything; don't understand what I'm doing. I've encountered this problem more with those who want just to hang on to their problems.

When I see the healing power taking hold in a person's energy field, and not being absorbed immediately, I know that the effects of my healing will be felt in a few days. 'That didn't work, I felt absolutely nothing,' they may say, only to find throughout the rest of the week their symptoms abating, their mood brightening and their humour returning.

I see people by appointment so I can give everyone time to allow them to pour out their troubles, especially if they have been through the mill and suffering for a long time with depression or panic attacks, or indeed are seriously ill and awaiting an operation.

One Friday morning the doorbell rang. A man in his early twenties hopped in on crutches, his right leg in plaster.

'I've just come in a taxi from the hospital,' he said. They're going to take me leg off! The doctors said gangrene has set in. They have to take the leg off!' he kept repeating – a look of terror on his face. John was his name. He was a musician in a well-known Irish band.

Late one night, after a gig, he accidentally put his foot through a plate-glass window, severing his Achilles' tendon in his right leg. They whisked him in an ambulance to hospital, screaming with pain. The doctors operated immediately – stitched the tendon together and encased his leg in plaster. John takes up the story:

'The next day, I was sent home on a pair of crutches, and told to keep the leg up. After a few hours, a strong throbbing sensation began in the leg – followed by this terrible stench. All my family and friends kept remarking on the terrible smell in the room. So I returned to the hospital the same day, and one of the doctors cut a porthole in the plaster, down to where the wound was. Fumes began to literally pour out through the hole – filling the whole place with a horrible stench. Two nurses had to run off and get a spray – to spray the whole ward. The doctor said the wound was badly infected. I was kept in the hospital for six weeks. They tried every form of medication, antibiotics, seaweed bandages, ulcer bandages, cancer dressings, etc. Nothing worked. They even tried doing a skin graft a number of times, but the infection was too bad.

For five months I went back and forth to the hospital, twice a day, to have it bandaged. The ward sister told me they had tried everything and nothing worked.

The head doctor then examined my leg and said the whole ankle was badly infected. Gangrene had set in. He told me, I might lose the leg.'

John broke down as he said the words '… lose the leg'. After a few minutes he composed himself and continued:

'The band I'm playing with is on a world tour and I haven't been able to work for over six months. I feel totally depressed about the whole thing. I just can't face losing me leg. They said they would go ahead with the operation on Monday. It's too unbelievable to even think about it.'

At that point it was time to do my stuff. I didn't have time to explain what I did or how it worked. John had a taxi waiting outside to bring him back to the hospital. I reached down to his leg and gave John as much healing as he could take through the plaster of Paris.

The surge of healing energy poured out my hands – right through the solid walls of the plaster and into the wound.

I transmitted more healing to his chest and head – to take away all the shock and trauma he was experiencing.

Monday morning, my doorbell rang. John came in smiling from ear to ear – no plaster of Paris, no crutches – just a limp. This was his experience of healing:

'When you put your hands on the plaster, Tony, I felt this tremendous heat coming from them. It went right through my Levi jeans, my thick sock, and through the plaster. It was as if you had a heater right up to my leg.

Then you put your hands on my chest, and back. At the time I was wearing a leather jacket, a thick Arran jumper and a T-shirt. The heat from your hands wasn't like an ordinary heat. I've often felt heat from my own hands. But this was a very strong intense heat flowing through me. It was a strange sensation coming from your hands – one I find hard to describe. But then when you put your hands on my head, it was spectacular. Everything began to spin, and I felt really high. When you finished, I remember trying to stand up, I just couldn't.

You grabbed a hold of me and got me to sit back down on the chair. After a few minutes, I burst out laughing. It was like

*laughing gas! I didn't walk out from your clinic – I floated out
on air.*

*When I arrived back at the hospital, the nurse who knew me
so well by now, commented on how much brighter I looked. So I
told her I'd been to see you for healing. I was taken aback when
she said, "That's who I would go to if I were sick." I got back
into the bed, and after about an hour the nurse opened the porthole in the plaster, and began shouting with excitement, "Look!
Look at the wound!" I couldn't see down the back of my leg, so
she ran off and returned with a mirror to show me. I looked
down at the leg reflected in the mirror. All the green stuff – all
the infection had gone. It had left a clean four to five-inch
wound, with a deep hole right into the bone. We watched as the
sides of the open wound came together, and gradually folded
over – just like pastry. We both kept looking at the wound, like
it was magic.*

*"I can't believe it!" the nurse kept saying. It was just amaz-
ing to watch. After that I was let home from the hospital and,
when I returned this morning, the doctor who has been dealing
with the case looked a bit puzzled as he examined the leg and
then said, "John, at long last your leg is healing." Then, as he
began cutting the plaster off, I looked over at the nurse and we
both smiled at each other.*

*As I was leaving the hospital, the nurse told me to come to
see you – to tell you what happened. I got a taxi home and got
on me bike and cycled all the way here this morning. It's a
bloody miracle.'*

John went off to New York, to catch up with his band on their
world tour. He returned to see me two months later. His limp had
gone, and he was in a buoyant mood. John fired a hundred-and-
one questions at me – about healing and why more people should
know about it.

The effects of healing can vary from person to person. Some get such a boost of energy they are 'raring to go'.

They want to get back into their lives – to catch up on all the things they were unable to do previously. I advise them to conserve their energy, to pace themselves, by doing a little at a time.

Years ago, when I first began healing, I remember a frail little lady in her seventies with cancer coming to see me. All she wanted healing for, she said, was to give her enough time to go to her solicitor and put her affairs in order. I gave her healing and off she went home.

'You never told me what was going to happen!' she said angrily, when she returned a week later.

'What's the matter?' I asked.

'Well, when I went home after seeing you I felt so much better. That night I went to sleep, delighted with myself.

The very next morning I bounced out of bed and took the whole house apart. I cleaned every room. I even took all the clothes out of presses for an airing; hoovered the house from top to bottom; tidied up the back garden, and washed my husband's car. I haven't done this in over twenty years.

When my husband came home from work, he said I'd gone mad. Derek, my son, said I was like someone plugged into the electric socket! After that I was finished, I felt completely exhausted, and fell into bed for three whole days. With all the energy I had, I felt I could tackle the whole world, but now I'm back to square one again.'

Others will feel the complete opposite. They need to go home and rest for a few hours. A great deal of healing has taken place on their physical counterpart – the aura. They feel sleepy and tired for a while, but then strengthen up and feel much better afterwards.

It wasn't all plain sailing trying to figure out how my gift worked. I remember an elderly man had come to see me. He was one of the early heart bypass patients in Ireland. He'd arrived with his wife, straight from his hospital bed, and wore pyjamas under his long trench coat. He suffered from severe pains in his ribs, he said. The wounds weren't healing very well.

Every time I went near him, beads of sweat broke out on his face. I had to stand a few feet away, out of range, until he calmed down. I tried several times to give him healing, but the same thing kept happening. Yet his wife was able to stand beside him perfectly well. At this stage I was getting worried.

I tuned in to my spirit friends for guidance. They told me that the energy fields around me were much too strong – I would need to take them down a step. I went away into the next room for a few minutes, and was shown how to visualise my energy fields, funnelling down into the ground. I went back into the room, with my energy on half-power. I was able to stand beside the man, put my hands on his chest and gave him healing.

When people come to see me suffering with an arthritic condition, I always suggest that they drink a few glasses of plain water after a healing session. This helps flush out the acid crystals that have been released from their joints as a result of the powerful healing energies stimulating their circulation. Similarly, if a patient has sinusitis, or is suffering with a chest condition, once healing had been absorbed, all the mucus and phlegm is released. A skin condition can become worse after healing. This is known as 'the healing crisis' and is only temporary. Then follows a dramatic improvement within twenty-four hours.

Over the years, the healing effects have surprised, baffled and amused both my patients and myself.

One of my patients, Rob, was a lead singer in a rock band, but he suffered with constant sore throats, which meant he was often unable to turn up for rehearsals. His voice was constantly irritated, dry and hoarse.

'We were supposed to be in Europe last week,' he whispered. 'The manager is going mad!'

The colours in his aura were dull, muddy and depleted, which told me he was burned out. When I put my hands to his throat he asked, 'Am I supposed to feel anything?'

'No,' I replied quickly, and continued with the healing.

'I didn't feel anything,' he whispered again, when I'd finished. But he made another appointment before he left.

I continued healing more people that morning, and at lunch-time went off for a bite to eat. As I reached my car, I saw him coming towards me through the crowd, beaming from ear to ear.

'As soon as I left you Tony, I went into the supermarket,' he said, his voice now good and strong. 'And as I got to the shelf with all the baked beans – I burst out laughing! I couldn't stop myself. The old women doing their shopping kept looking at me. The more I laughed – the more they laughed! So I ran around to the bread counter, breaking my sides laughing. Everywhere I went, these women kept following me, I was like the pied piper. The more I laughed – the more they laughed.

'Eventually I had to come out of the shop. Tony, is this supposed to happen?' he grinned and continued breaking his sides laughing!

I always recommend to everyone coming for the first time to leave any preconceived ideas or notions outside the door. Over the years I have heard some strange and sometimes daft ideas about healing.

A middle-aged woman came to see me dressed from head to toe in deep purple. I thought she was going to a rock concert! She was wearing a purple dress, a purple blouse and purple shoes. Her handbag and her fingernails were purple. When she sat down she let out a deep sigh and turned to me and said, 'I hope this is the right colour to wear for healing.'

Another woman looked very uncomfortable, sitting in the chair with her handbag on her lap. I was just about to give her healing when she hauled out of her bag a large amethyst crystal stone, about the size of a flower pot.

'There – that's much better,' she exclaimed as she plonked the heavy stone on to my desk.

'I've been carrying that stone with me all day in me bag. It weighs a bloody ton,' she said as she drew breath and continued. 'I was told it would help protect me against negative and evil forces when you're healing me.' Then she looked at me as if to say, 'So – what are you waiting for …?'

Other such notions can be more damaging. One morning as I was healing I felt a strange feeling coming from the waiting room. Everyone seemed to be very obedient and on their best behaviour. After the sixth patient came through the door I asked a young woman with asthma if something was wrong. She looked carefully over her shoulder and lowered her voice to a whisper and said, 'While I was sitting in your waiting room chatting, a woman who was in earlier told me I could only come three times. She said, "If the healing doesn't work, it's because you're meant to be ill – it's your punishment from God."'

Unfortunately, this brand of negativity has been doing the rounds for quite some time.

There are those who will come just once, out of curiosity. Their minds are closed to receiving any form of help. I believe that whatever attitude you come with that's exactly what you'll find.

Some want me to convince them to come again. This immediately sets up the wrong chemistry. There has to be trust and openness between the patient and healer. The golden rule is that healing is offered, it's never imposed.

Perhaps one of the greatest misconceptions about spiritual healing is that miracles occur all the time. This is not the case in practice. More often than not there is a gradual improvement. As the old saying goes:

We don't get ill overnight.
We don't get better overnight.
It takes time.

When someone with severe arthritis comes to see me, for example, they may find they are taking fewer painkillers over time. They are able to climb the stairs more easily, or take up the hoover and clean the house.

A patient *can* experience instantaneous healing. This is wonderful for them and their family when it happens. However, it's not always the rule. Progress is more usually gradual and results are seen over a longer period of time. At times there can be setbacks – symptoms of flu, relationship difficulties or problems in the work place – all can be a major factor in making a full recovery.

I have seen many a patient who had been making good steady progress, when they experienced a sudden death in the family. This leaves them badly shaken. Their symptoms then flare up once more, leaving them despondent and depressed. It takes time and lots of loving care to get them back on their feet again.

Many patients have also told me of their disappointment on seeing other healers, and not being cured. Yet nobody would expect an instant cure from their doctor. A chronic condition may have taken many years to develop, for example chronic eczema, a hiatus hernia or a weeping leg ulcer. All of these can take weeks, months or longer to heal fully.

In order to give healing a fair chance to work, I always recommend that the patient comes to me for six visits; to see how their condition responds to my healing treatment. At each visit, I monitor the positive effects so both of us can see clearly the progress made.

Sometimes, I am asked to heal the impossible. For that reason I cannot promise a cure, any more than a doctor can. The physical body may have broken down to a point where the healing cannot stimulate a complete response. Yet there can be many other bene-fits to be received for that person.

I try to suspend any negative ideas I may have as to the outcome. If a miracle occurs – then it's that person's time to be healed. It's taken me years to accept this part of my gifts and let whatever happens, happen.

Jim was working as a carpenter when he was struck down with crip-pling arthritis. At that point his life came to an abrupt stop. All medical treatment had ceased:

'Good health was something I always took for granted until I was diagnosed as having that dreaded illness called rheumatoid arthritis; a diagnosis itself that took many months of exhaust-ing clinical tests, pain and misery, and a lengthy stay in hospi-tal for treatment. I wasn't in hospital very long before I realised that there was no cure for this progressively crippling disease. All one could hope for, was that some time in the future some scien-tist would find a permanent, non-toxic, non-addictive drug, a drug that would not be withdrawn for reasons of public safety, as in the case of some recent disclosures. Upon my discharge from hospital in a wheelchair and clinging to my bottle of tablets I could still hear the social worker's voice ringing in my ear, telling me I would have to face reality that I could no longer continue in my physically active job. She said she would help fix me up in a sheltered workshop.

You can well imagine the depressed state I now found myself in; twenty-seven years old with a young family and little hope for the future, until by providence I met a girl who told me about you, Tony, and the remarkable results she herself had obtained. Needless to say I presented myself at your healing clinic, and to my good fortune you were conducting a healing session. I explained my condition and I can honestly say that you were the first person who knew how I felt, and who could offer any hope of improvement. In your own way you set about it immediately. Every day I felt better; the dreadful pain was gone. In the space of two months I came from a depressed, painful existence into one of active participation in rebuilding my life. It is now twenty years since I met you, Tony, and it's a pleasure to thank you publicly for not only ridding me of the pain and discomfort and curing my arthritis, but also for guiding me towards a new way of life.'

People often ask me 'if they need to have faith' in order for healing to work. The simple answer is no. Whether the person believes or not has never hampered my ability to heal them. Children, babies and animals are oblivious to the notion of faith, yet I have healed them. Another good example is healing from a distance – called absent healing. The person is unaware that healing has been sought on their behalf. Yet the healing has worked. 'Faith and belief' are just labels put on healing down through the years, which only serve to confuse people.

Then there is the sceptical patient who has been browbeaten into coming: Joe walked through my door one day, having suffered for several years with ulcerative colitis, a chronic inflammatory disease of the large intestine and rectum.

'I don't want to waste your time!' was the first thing he said as he stood outside my door. 'I've only come because Tommy, a chap I used to work with, drops into me flat to see how I am doing. I've had more arguments with him!

'He keeps pestering me to come and see you. I keep telling him I can't be cured but he keeps saying, "Joe! You could be the one in a million!"

'To get him off my back – would you tell him I've been to see you?' he pleaded before turning on his heels to go.

'Tell me what the problem is,' I asked.

'Colitis! I've got colitis. I'm taking loads of steroids every day. There is no cure. I've been on the hospital waiting list for two years now. I suppose they're busy in the hospital.'

'I urged him to come in and sit down,' but Joe kept repeating, 'I've got to go now!'

Eventually after much persuasion he came in to my room and nervously sat on the chair.

Just as I began to explain what I did, he burst out with, 'I'm not here for that! I don't believe in anything like that. Just tell Tommy when you see him that I came.' He went to get up off the chair, so I quickly changed the subject and asked what he worked at.

'I used to work in a hotel in town. But I can't now. I haven't worked in about three years since the illness. I won't ever work again, it's over for me,' he said with a deep sadness in his voice.

'I haven't been able to go outside the flat. The weight's fallen off me. I had to come here by taxi.'

'What do you do in your flat all day?' I enquired.

'Read books – look out the window at the traffic going by. That's all I can do. Forty years of age and I'll never work again. I don't have any energy any more, all my leg muscles have gone, there's no power in them.' His upset showed as he hung his head and stared at the floor. A moment later he got up off the chair and headed for the door.

'Sit down please,' I urged once again.

Reluctantly he sat down and started talking about his deceased parents. I reached out and put my hands on his stomach.

'What are you doing?'

'I'm giving you healing.'

'I don't want anything! I haven't come for anything. I don't believe in anything like this,' he protested.

It was too late. The healing power had already flowed through my hands into his stomach. Joe suddenly stopped talking and went very quiet.

'What's that coming from your hands?' he asked.

'It's the healing power. Can you feel it?'

'Yes! It's like a mild tingling going through me.'

'That's it! That's exactly what it is,' I said while moving my hands from place to place.

Slowly a smile crossed Joe's face. He jumped up on his feet and began rubbing his stomach. 'The pain's gone!' he shouted. 'It's gone!'

His whole face lit up. Excitement grew in his voice; one smile followed another as he rubbed his stomach.

Joe kept me for an hour that day, talking all about healing, how it worked and quizzing me about my life. It was one of those magic moments.

The following week Joe arrived back for another appointment. He looked a different man.

'After being with you, Tony, I ate everything – everything I couldn't eat before,' he said, smiling from ear to ear.

'Cornflakes, beans on toast, all kinds of fruit. I've even went to the local chipper and had fish and chips. On the weekend I borrowed a bicycle and cycled out to the seaside, about fifteen miles away, and got in for a dip!

'I've managed to cycle up the mountains a few times even though I lost a lot of muscle in my legs. It's unbelievable! I still can't believe it,' he kept saying as I healed him some more.

'Will you thank Tommy – the chap that sent you?' I asked as he sailed out the door.

'I will, Tony! I will,' he promised as he whistled down the stairs.

After a few visits, Joe took his name off the waiting list and went back to work – a new man.

Some find it difficult to equate the effectiveness of healing with their idea of 'logic'. They are used to seeing everything from a tablet and medical point of view.

'Maybe it was the steroid cream?' asked a woman whose psoriasis had suddenly vanished.

'And how long have you been using the creams?' I asked.

'Oh – five or six years now.'

'My back and hips feel better. I think it's because the weather has suddenly got that bit warmer,' another reasoned.

'Well, when the weather gets colder, and if you remain pain-free, perhaps you'll consider the effects of healing.'

A woman who was suffering with irritable bowel syndrome came to see me recently. For over thirty years she had felt nothing but severe pain, chronic depression, dizziness and mood swings. I could see how distressed she was, so I listened to her story and said little.

When I gave her healing, the healing power flowed through her with ease. She commented that she could feel electricity coming from my hands and moving around her body. On her second appointment she looked so much better. Her symptoms had all gone she said. She had the best pain-free week in many years. The transformation was amazing. She turned to me and said, 'At long last the tablets are beginning to work …!'

Most people, however, once they start getting well, want to know more. At that point I can answer their questions and give them some advice on how they can help themselves.

Then there are those who simply can't acknowledge an improvement, for fear their illness may return.

Anne, a mother of two, suffered each day with blinding, severe migraine headaches. On her third visit for healing, she gave me a piece of paper, which read: 'I am feeling so much better now, thank you. It's been the best three weeks of my life.'

At the bottom of the page she concluded: 'I don't want to say it out loud, for fear of flying in the face of God.'

This I call 'the Irish guilt syndrome'. Many are burdened with these terrible feelings of guilt, fearful of saying anything good about themselves. Uncovering and releasing this guilt is like freeing a trapped bird from its cage.

Julie was suffering with a very bad circulation problem in her left leg. In fact it was completely numb – from her hip to her big toe. She had already been to various hospitals and doctors for all the usual tests and treatments. She tried acupuncture, reflexology and many other therapies, but nothing seemed to work. Julie described how she had little or no feeling in her left leg. It was completely frozen and numb.

Sure enough, when I reached down and placed my hands on her leg it was like a solid block of ice. The healing power flowed from my hands; Julie couldn't feel a thing. She just looked at me strangely. Undaunted, I continued tuning in to her, and asked my spirit friends for help.

Immediately, an impression of a tall man formed in my mind's eye. I looked at Julie and asked, 'How is your father?'

There was complete silence. Julie stared at me.

'I really don't know what this has got to do with my leg,' she replied curtly.

'Is he dead? Is your father dead?' I asked once more.

While I waited for a reply, Julie sat stone-faced.

'I really don't understand what it's got to do with my leg!' she insisted.

A part of me wanted 'to be let off the hook', but I was urged on by my spirit friends.

'I'm just wondering what sort of a man your father was,' I probed further.

'Oh. He died a few years ago!' Julie snapped.

'What happened to him?' I asked.

'It's odd that you ask that question,' she said finally. Her tone changed to a softer pitch.

'My dad died in hospital only hours after he had his leg amputated.'

'Which leg was it?' I enquired.

Julie thought deeply for a moment then put her hand on her left leg and said, 'That's funny. My father had the problem in his left leg. The same as mine.'

'How long ago did your father pass away?' I asked.

Julie let out a deep sigh. Tears welled up in her eyes.

'I used to be awake every night, in the bedroom next door, listening to him screaming with the pain in his leg,' she said, her voice shaking. 'Gangrene set in and he had to go to hospital. He died the next day after having his leg amputated. It was seven years ago!' she cried.

'How long have you had this problem with your leg?' I quietly asked.

A look of surprise came across her face.

'It's about seven years now,' she said.

I smiled as Julie made the connection.

'You ...You ... don't think that ...?' she stammered.

'Yes, I do,' I replied. 'After the dreadful shock you experienced with your dad, the power in your leg switched off. You tried to take away his pain.'

Julie broke down and sobbed her heart out. When she had emptied all the upset that had been buried deep within – the life flowed back into her leg again. Her trauma had finally been removed.

One day, when I looked into the waiting room, my eye fixed on a tall young man in his thirties, seated among four women and a young child. He wore a pair of white tennis shorts, flip flops and a white short-sleeved vest. The women chatted around the heater, in their warm overcoats. It was the middle of November, and the temperature outside was two degrees below zero.

'It's OK, Tony,' said one of the women next in line. 'I think this man is next.'

Everyone could see how poorly the man was. He stood up and

waddled slowly behind me into my healing room. Sitting carefully on the edge of the chair, he introduced himself as Patrick. As he explained in a low painful voice that he was an accountant by profession, I could see he was covered from head to toe in weeping eczema. He had suffered with this condition for the past twelve years now, he said. He had been out of work for the last three-and-a-half years, unable to put clothes on to go out. His small, depleted, silvery-grey aura that barely glowed around his body told me that his whole system had completely broken down. As he struggled to catch his next breath, I could also see that he was suffering with asthma, which he forgot to mention.

Patrick sat uncomfortably in front of me. He was over six foot tall, very thin, half-naked and his skin weeping fluid from all directions. With his legs wide apart he deliberately kept his arms extended from his body. He kept all his fingers apart, his hands in mid-air hovering a few inches over his weeping knees.

He had four matchsticks neatly wrapped in cotton wool between each of his toes to keep them apart. His long, wispy hair was flattened and glued to his head.

He was afraid to sit back on the chair, for fear that his short vest might get stuck to his body. As he spoke, the glue-like substance poured from his roaring red skin – down his face, arms and legs. His eyelids began to stick together as he struggled to blink his eyes. Every few moments he would reach down to the floor and take out a fresh handkerchief from a plastic bag to dab his eyes. Patrick was a sight to behold.

'I've been to everyone and anyone,' he said as he struggled with a dreadful wheeze, gasping for more air. 'I can't even go outside the door. All day I have to sit completely naked with just a small towel wrapped around me. Three years ago, my girlfriend and I bought a house together – thinking we might get married, but I can't now. I've been living on my own in the new house.

'It looks like I'll spend the rest of my life there – on my own,' he said as tears filled his eyes.

'As for my work, three years ago I was in the process of being made a partner in the business – now that looks like it's never going to happen. It's so depressing. I don't think my girlfriend will stay around much longer the way things are.'

'How do you go to sleep at night?' I asked.

'I leave it as late as I can. I try to sleep sitting up on a hard sofa with nothing over me,' he explained.

'The worst is the next morning. My eyelids are always glued together. I got a bottle of this stuff from the hospital. I pour it on some cotton wool, and rub it over my eyelids. It can take about twenty minutes to work and eventually when one eyelid is free, I can see around the room and work from there. Different parts of my body are usually stuck together – so it can take a few hours to completely free myself.'

By now the backs of Patrick's legs were sticking to the chair. He had to stand up and walk slowly around the room. His wheezing grew louder with the intense effort.

When he sat back down, I wasted no time and tried to give him healing, but there was nowhere to place my hands. The watery green substance flowed down his whole body. So I held my hands a few inches away, just touching the edge of his energy field. As the healing energies flowed into his chest the terrible wheezing began to ease. When I got to the energy field around his head, my hands seemed to flow right into his mind. I could feel the extreme terror and trauma he was feeling, and sought healing from my spirit friends to help take it all away.

Within moments, the dark bank of cloud lifted, revealing a brighter energy field beneath. When the healing power stopped flowing, I told Patrick it would take six months to free him of his misery.

'I don't care how long it takes. I'm not going anywhere,' he replied nervously.

Patrick arrived every week for healing. As his skin began to heal, he'd wear a new piece of clothing each visit. Soon he was able to wear a short-sleeved shirt; another day he wore a pair of trousers. Eventually he turned up in a navy blue suit, shirt, tie, socks and shoes, to the applause from some people he got to know in the waiting room. He resumed his life and went back to work. On his final visit, he shook my hands warmly and announced, 'I'm getting married next week, Tony. Wish me luck.'

EXERCISE – THE HEALING BREATH

One of the best ways to open the channels within yourself for healing is to practise the following simple breathing exercise:

- Sitting on a comfortable chair, close your eyes and be aware of your breath. Whenever possible, breathe in through your nose and out through your nose.
- Follow your breath as it flows into your lungs and then flows out again.
- Now let your breath become slow and deep. Breathe right down into your tummy.
- Imagine as you breathe in you are breathing in white light and as you breathe out you are breathing out all the dark colours trapped in your body.
- You can now concentrate this light to wherever you feel unwell.

CHAPTER 5

AURAS

'Your Aura is the key to your real self. It is the visible expression of your mind, soul and spirit. The condition of your aura depends on whether you are experiencing the light within.'

S.G.J. Ousley

Muriel, a tall, slim woman in her early forties, sat crouched on the edge of the chair, her chest rasping as she struggled to breathe. Her face looked pale and withdrawn with dark rings under her eyes. Muriel rummaged through her handbag scattering a colourful array of tablets and inhalers to the floor. She stared at me anxiously – her eyes pleading for help.

When I looked at her aura I could see a solid block of dark green pressing down on her chest. The colour green meant Muriel was 'a giver' – that she gave with a heart-and-a-half. Yet this compressed energy stuck in and around her heart chakra was more revealing; it told me she was deeply heart-broken. No sooner had I closed my eyes and placed my hands on her shoulders than I felt the familiar healing energies flowing down through me. Minutes later, a calmness enveloped her.

She let out a deep sigh and began to relax. The wheezing in her chest softened. All her anxiety and fear ebbed slowly away. I felt her sit upright immediately I took my hands away. Muriel had changed before my eyes. The colour had come back into her cheeks. She was no longer struggling to breathe. I pulled up a chair and asked what had happened to her.

Muriel told me she had had a good job in the bank, but had to give it up to nurse her husband, Jim, who'd died from cancer seven years earlier. She cared for him for two solid years, while rearing her two young girls, all on her own. 'That's when the asthma kicked in,' she explained. Muriel told me how she used numerous inhalers and steroids each day, spending most of her time in bed and following a ritual of antibiotic courses, one after the other. But nothing helped. When she had finished I explained to her about the congestion I saw in her aura around her chest and heart area. I asked had she ever been able to cry.

'Cry?!' she said angrily. 'For years psychologists and psychiatrists have suggested to me I try different things to make myself cry. I just can't tell you how many weepy films I've been to. I've chopped onions to beat the band – I've even tried putting pepper up my nose – but nothing's worked! I hope you're not going to tell me to do the same?' she asked despondently.

I assured her I wouldn't recommend any such foolishness. Over the years I've heard all kinds of daft suggestions by these so-called experts. Instead I gave Muriel more healing to unblock the energy channels around her lungs and heart chakra, to help boost her depleted system. On her second visit she returned, looking radiant. This was Muriel's experience of healing:

'When I arrived home that morning, after seeing you Tony, I'd just turned the key in the door, when suddenly I burst out crying – something I hadn't been able to do since my Jim died. I ran up the stairs to my bedroom and wept and wept – I couldn't hold the tears back. I used up every tissue and handkerchief in the house.

When my daughters arrived home from school, they asked me to promise I would never see 'that terrible man' again, who'd upset their mother so. I cried non-stop for three continuous days.

Look at the skin on my face!

It's all broken out in a rash from constantly drying my tears.
I've used up every towel in the house. It's just bloody marvellous,
Tony! You know, I've been playing tennis all week with my
friends – something I hadn't been able to do for years. I can at
last breathe again, it's just wonderful.'

Most problems show up in the first three auras; and these are the ones
I mainly work with. The first is the etheric aura, known as the physical
aura, which surrounds the whole body. The second is the emotional
aura, which is focused through the solar plexus, just above the navel.
The third is the mental aura, which surrounds the head.

When there is a disturbance of any kind in these energy fields,
the result is often ill health in the physical body. What we experience as tension in the stomach, for example, is in fact a ball of
congested energy trapped in and around the solar plexus.

If I place my hands on this area and channel the healing energies
into the solar plexus, the congestion will soon break up and disperse.

Very often I'm boosting a depleted system. The weak colours in
the aura will look fused together, appearing watery and white-
washed. After a healing treatment, these colours begin to separate
out and regain their vibrancy.

When there is an overload in the emotional aura, owing to a shock
of some kind or from suppressing one's feelings – the aura appears as
if it's bulging out and down one side of the body. For this I will put
my hand on to the emotional chakra in the solar plexus and run
energy through it to clear out the stress. Once the emotional aura
frees out it appears to glow evenly around the body.

YOUR ENERGY SYSTEM AND HOW IT WORKS

To understand about your own aura and how it functions
you must first think in terms of energy. When you turn on your

television set, the electricity passes through various conductors, giving life to pictures and sound.

Your aura or energy system is similar. It is made up of streams of coloured light that flow from your soul, weaving together to form your spiritual, mental, emotional and physical life.

Each stream of coloured light passes through a conductor or prism known as 'chakras', which give life through the seven major glands in your physical body. Each chakra radiates its own individual colour – red, orange, green etc. – right through the colour spectrum to white, just like the rainbow.

All together there are seven major chakras, each a blueprint of the seven major endocrine glands. They exist on the etheric level, etheric meaning the state between energy and matter, and are situated along the central axis of the spinal cord, called the 'Sushumna' in Sanskrit.

The word chakra, pronounced 'Chak-ra', is an ancient Sanskrit word meaning 'wheels of light'. Universal energies, or the life force, flow through these wheels and make them spin.

When spinning they look like sparklers or spinning tops, constantly drawing in life force from the universe into their energy counterpart. When a chakra is below par, the corresponding energy field or aura will look weak or absent.

When a person is healthy, the chakras will spin clockwise, drawing in the correct amount of energy from the universe. Under stress, however, the chakras spin anti-clockwise, and lose energy; the physical system is left weak and depleted.

THE FIRST CHAKRA – RED AURA

The first chakra relates to the first light energy body, also called the etheric aura. The etheric aura is an exact blueprint of our physical body. It has all the anatomical parts of the physical body and looks rather like a delicate spider's web. This web supports the life force that feeds vitality and nourishment into our muscles, cells and organs.

This first chakra is linked to the gonadic system, the reproduction process, sexual functioning and physical energy. The colour vibration in the aura is red. It relates to the physical dimension – the basic symbol of life. Red in a person's aura can signify passion, anger, wilfulness, excitement, aggression, jealousy, impulsiveness, restlessness, nervousness and temper.

When a person has poor healing or circulation problems, for example, it is this chakra that is not functioning properly. During a healing treatment, I will transmit the red healing rays of energy into the first chakra and to the problem area. Many will experience heat coming from my hands passing through them as the healing treatment takes effect.

When anger is bottled up and not expressed, this red energy accumulates in the etheric aura, and pockets itself somewhere within the physical body.

The result can be a whole range of inflammatory problems: raging headaches, stomach ulcers, back problems, eruptions, digestive problems, pain, hypertension and numerous skin conditions.

Henrietta was a prim, silver-haired woman in her seventies and, as she sat across the room from me in her sensible tweeds and with a walking cane, I was reminded of Agatha Christie's genteel sleuth, Miss Marple.

'I was in a bad car crash, and ended up in hospital for over a year-and-a-half,' she sighed, while struggling to get comfortable in the chair. 'They tried everything, but nothing eases the damn pain!'

She was suffering with a very painful back and hip condition, she said, which affected her ability to stand, sit or walk. Well – that's the practical explanation! I told myself. However, as I looked at her aura I could see it was shot through with streaks of red – she was holding in lots of anger.

I asked if somebody had upset her in the past, someone she was still angry with.

Henrietta looked at me with a note of surprise as if I had turned a key and discovered her well-hidden secret. Then she told me of a neighbour who'd regularly given her a lift to the shops in her car until one day they were in a bad crash – her neighbour came away without a scratch – but she ended up in hospital.

'You know, Tony, all the time I was there, she never came to see me. When I came out of the hospital, my poor husband, Tom, nursed me and not once did she darken my door. Before the crash, she would drop in on us at any time to share a cup of tea and a chat,' she said resentfully, her angry voice filling the room.

'Maybe she blamed herself for causing the accident?' I suggested. But the woman wouldn't listen, she kept going on and on about how dreadful the neighbour was.

'Could you possibly forgive her?' I asked.

'How? How can I forgive her!' she protested. 'The woman died five years ago!'

At first I thought she was joking. Then I realised I'd neglected to ask when the accident had occurred.

With some words of advice about forgiveness, I gave her healing to help remove the anger. On her next appointment, Henrietta told me she had lit a candle in the church for the neighbour and forgave her. That night she noticed that all the pain had gone from her back and hips and legs; she got her best night's sleep in years. The transformation was amazing. All the pain had completely disappeared – so, too, had all the angry red streaks in her aura.

THE SECOND CHAKRA – ORANGE AURA

The second chakra is located around the pancreas centre. This centre houses the emotions, and shows up in the aura as the colour vibration orange. From here are expressed feelings and emotions, sensitivity and 'gut feeling'.

This emotional body is lighter than the etheric body. It extends to about three-and-a-half inches beyond the physical body. As the emotions constantly shift and change, the pattern of colours within the aura changes accordingly. Dark and muddy colours, for instance, tell me that old stuff is bottled up from the past.

Suppressing emotions can cause various mental problems, such as depression, panic attacks and low self-esteem.

With shock, the emotional aura expands, fragmenting a few feet from the body. There, the colours steadily drain, the energy field looks pale, milky and lifeless. The aura then compresses into the physical body, absorbing all the shock, deep into the nervous system where the emotional chakra lies. The person feels numb, drained of all energy and is left in a fog of depression.

Healing is wonderful for getting rid of shock; it immediately frees out the stress and disturbance in the emotional chakra. This causes the aura to 'spring' back out again, radiating its vibrant, healthy orange glow.

Golden orange reflects vitality, strength, optimism and good humour. When a person is feeling repressed, dissatisfied, insecure, lacking ambition and control, the aura reflects a dark orange, streaked with red. The person may seek refuge in overeating – in an attempt to fill up the emptiness they feel inside.

When encountering fear or panic, the aura turns a dark, mauvey orange. This is experienced as a tense feeling in the pit of the stomach, where the emotional chakra lies.

When there is a predominance of orange in the aura, a person may be egotistical and self-centred. I frequently see an abundance of orange in the auras of teenagers and students.

THE THIRD CHAKRA – YELLOW AURA

The third chakra relates to the mental aura, located in the area of the solar plexus just above the emotional centre. This chakra is linked to the adrenal glands and nervous system. The colour vibration is yellow, and radiates three to seven inches beyond the physical body. Contained within the mental aura is a spectrum of intellectual thoughts and ideas.

Just as the emotional aura expands and contracts, as feelings and experiences change, so, too, does the mental aura. When a person feels stressed-out, for example, a pale, weak yellow will show up in the mental aura.

If someone is mentally negative or depressed, the aura will look dark, depleted and withdrawn – a mere glimmer around the head. Confused thinking shows up as blobs of grey, pulsating slowly through the yellow aura. When a person is positive and happy, the mental aura looks bright and vibrant, pulsating around the head and shoulders.

This chakra also has to do with the intellect and linear mind. When functioning correctly, the colour in the aura is a vibrant yellow – the person is mentally active, quick thinking, intelligent, stable and reliable. However, when the yellow is weak or pale, the person tends to daydream and let others make decisions for them.

When I see auras that are completely yellow and devoid of all other colour, this tells me that the person is living theoretically – in their head. They've cut off their emotions, and are living life purely as a mental exercise. I've treated many a marriage crisis, where one partner is living their married life with such a rigid mind set. The same can be said of someone who's overly intellectual; whose mind is constantly 'chattering', like a broken record. This person finds it almost impossible to break free from this constant chatter and is, in effect, a prisoner of their own mind.

THE FOURTH CHAKRA – GREEN AURA

The first three chakras are called the 'lower centres' because they relate to basic human nature. The fourth chakra, however, is seen as one of the higher spiritual centres; often referred to as the gateway to the spirit, or soul. This chakra radiates the colour green and is connected to the thymus gland, the lungs and the heart.

Located in the centre of the chest, it's known as the chakra of love, healing and compassion.

In the physical body, the thymus deals with the lympathic system, the immune system, healing and fighting off infection. A healthy green radiation from this chakra means the healing mechanism is functioning correctly. Green in the aura indicates a person who is reliable, trustworthy, helpful, friendly and a 'rock of good sense'. Those who possess the healing gift function from the heart centre and have green radiating in their aura.

The heart chakra is your very own personal healer. When you have stressful thoughts and emotions, it helps keep your energy channels clear. Green is also the colour of Mother Nature, and nature can have a powerful healing influence on the whole being. When you feel stressed-out, for example, a long walk in the countryside, breathing in the fresh air, can help revive you and problems just seem to melt away. This is Mother Nature at work, healing, clearing away all negativity from the energy fields.

When a sympathetic friend listens and gives advice from the heart, this person has green radiating in their aura. Similarly, a person with green fingers will inspire even the most difficult plants to grow, and revive those that are wilting or dying. Such a person has their heart chakra open; they project love to their plants, just like a mother pours love and nourishment from her heart to her child.

I've known healers who were excellent at treating physical problems such as shingles, arthritis, ringworm and gout. But when it came to the mind, emotional and psychic areas, success eluded them. This is because they had not developed their gift fully through the other chakras and as a result were only putting out the physical energies.

Part of spiritual development – the journey through life – is to experience pure love, from the heart. Sadly, many people are told at an early age that to love oneself is selfish. This belief causes so much damage. They are left cut off from this nourishment from their spirit that is there waiting to be tapped into.

When two people fall in love, fine strings of etheric energy bind one heart chakra to another. This is also true of the emotional and mental chakras; both are on the same wavelength, as it were. If the relationship breaks up, I see a severing of these energy strings. The partners are left 'broken-hearted'. The same can be said of a person who's lost a partner in life through bereavement; their heart strings are broken. There's a void, an emptiness felt deep within.

A depressed person may experience the same feelings of emptiness as someone who is bereaved. Each mourns the lack of close contact with their higher selves – their spirit.

THE FIFTH CHAKRA – BLUE AURA

The fifth chakra is linked to the thyroid gland in the throat, and radiates the colour blue in the aura. On the physical level, the thyroid gland controls the nervous system, temperature, metabolism and energy. On the spiritual level, the fifth chakra is where higher thoughts are formed and relates to the creative mind, self-confidence, inspiration and will-power.

If you have an inspired 'creative flash' or 'revelation', this means you are tapping into this level of consciousness. Many of the great philosophers, inventors, artists, poets and musicians have been inspired by this inner voice. Some heard poetry or music, while others had visions either when awake or through dreaming.

Those with blue in their auras are often inspired by a higher purpose and some are dedicated to the work of community service. They are natural born leaders, and possess the will to get things done.

The fifth chakra is connected to the throat, and it's from here people express themselves. If someone feels tongue-tied, unable to say how they feel, the throat chakra is blocked. This blockage can manifest itself as a sore throat, swollen glands, inflamed vocal chords, loss of voice or stammer.

When a light blue is reflected in the aura, it means that the person is searching for a meaning to life. This can take them down a religious path. If the blue is lighter still, the person is weak-willed, shallow, melancholic and struggling with problems. 'In the blues' or 'feeling blue' means that the throat chakra is out of balance. A deep blue in the aura, however, shows that the person has arrived, spiritually, at their destination.

THE SIXTH CHAKRA – VIOLET AURA

The sixth chakra relates to the pineal gland. It radiates through the aura as the colour violet. Located at the centre of the upper part of the head, just above the pituitary gland, it's the chakra of the upper brain – the cerebrum.

It draws life force to the front part of the brain, and when violet is pulsating through the aura, it can mean the person is psychic and has universal awareness. The person knows that they are part of a greater will and they can see beyond this material life.

THE SEVENTH CHAKRA – WHITE AURA

The seventh chakra is linked to the pituitary gland, often referred to as the master gland, because it controls the other six major endocrine glands. This chakra draws in life force to the lower brain – the cerebellum.

Located in the centre of the forehead, between the two eyes, it is commonly known as 'the third eye'. In ancient times it was called the 'eye of light' or the 'eye of spirit' – symbolising the connection between man and God. This aura is our spirit aura, and contains all the other auras. Extending two to three feet out beyond the physical body, it radiates as the colour white, almost a silvery white.

THE SHAPE OF THE AURA

The shape of an aura, however, can be as important as its colour – take the example of a young woman who walked into my healing room. Immediately my eyes were riveted on what seemed like two cement blocks at her feet. Her aura 'bulged' below her knees. From her waist to her head and shoulders, her aura was sucked in, like clingfilm. Her energy chakras were sluggishly spinning, like windmills with no wind to power them.

'I feel stuck!' she cried. 'As if I'm stuck to the ground. Nothing's moving in my life. I've no friends. No relationships. I keep getting stuck in dead-end jobs.'

Nothing was moving in her life, because her aura was literally down at her feet. She had cut herself off from the brighter side of her mind and emotions.

The opposite of this is the mushroom-shaped aura. It's big on top, then narrows at the bottom. This person is using their mind to dominate. They're big into power play by taking advantage of others.

The unstable aura shoots out in all directions. As the mind and emotions constantly change, so, too, does the shape of the aura.

A withdrawn aura looks like a plastic bag, sucked of air. The seven chakras are barely moving. The person feels powerless to effect any change in their life.

Some people can drain others of energy. They're what I call 'energy vampires'. Their aura looks as if it has hooks, almost like tentacles, coming out from the head and solar plexus. When you come into contact with them, their auric energies, being low or depleted, will rise. They feel good in your company. However, your energy levels will gradually drop, leaving you completely drained and exhausted.

EXERCISES – SEEING AURAS

The four exercises that follow will help you to practise seeing auras.

EXERCISE 1

❧ Get an indoor castor oil or peace-lily plant. Place it on a table close to a white background – a bright wall will do. Relax in a chair and stare at one of the leaves for a few minutes. Look to a quarter-of-an-inch beyond the edge of the leaf. Now slowly move your eyes up and down the edge of the leaf, and just beyond it.

❦ Look for a very fine pencil line, running just off the edge of the leaf. This is the etheric aura; the physical life force aura of the plant.

EXERCISE 2

❦ Place your hand over a white sheet of paper. Look at your fore-finger, then out beyond its edge for a few minutes. The fine pencil line you see at the edge of your finger is your etheric aura – the life force aura in your body.

EXERCISE 3

❦ Bring the tip of your forefinger right up to the edge of the plant. Can you see both auras? Bring them closer until they touch. Sometimes the plant reacts by flickering and moving slightly. When this happens you've effectively sparked energy from your finger's aura, to the plant's aura.

EXERCISE 4

❦ Look in a mirror and try to see your aura. First place a white background behind you and gaze slowly into the mirror from one shoulder to the other.

❦ Look to about a quarter-of-an-inch beyond the outline of your body. With practice you will be surprised to see your own etheric aura.

With further practice you will be able to see colours in your aura. Write down the colours you have seen, and look back through the list of colours and their meaning as described in this chapter. This will tell you how your health energy is, and what mental emotional and spiritual levels you are expressing yourself from.

CHAPTER 6

HEALING CHILDREN

'The future belongs to those who believe in the beauty of their dreams.'

Eleanor Roosevelt.

E VER SINCE STEVEN SPIELBERG made the film *E.T.* my job as a healer has been so much easier – especially where children are concerned. There's a scene in the film where the alien's friend and protector, the little boy Elliot, cuts his finger and it starts to bleed. Seeing his little friend in trouble, E.T. raises his forefinger towards the sky and it lights up like a beacon. Rays of wondrous light pour from the finger. E.T. places it gently on to Elliot's wound. Energy jumps from one finger to another and the little boy's wound heals over immediately. Elliot is stunned, but smiling with awe and delight. Children who've seen the film accept healing just as Elliot did.

Some children suffer with physical and mental illnesses, the very same as adults, but they can't express it as clearly as an adult can. It's always been easy for me to tune in to a child's world, to discover where their true problem lies.

I've treated hundreds of children who were bullied at school, for example, long before the problem of bullying became recognised like it is today.

'Paul keeps getting nose-bleeds,' his mother said. 'Each morning it happens I have to take him straight away to the hospital. It's been going on for months now! The doctors are fed up cauterising his bloodied nose.'

Paul, aged nine, was bunched up in the chair holding a handkerchief to his nose.

'I bet he doesn't get them on a Saturday or Sunday,' I said as I tuned in to him.

'No!' she said thoughtfully. 'No, he doesn't seem to. Why is that?'

'How are you getting on in school?' I asked Paul.

'I hate it. I hate it, hate it!' he choked. 'Everyone bullies me. It's just not fair!'

'It's certainly news to me,' his astonished mother said.

After one healing session and some practical advice, Paul never suffered from a nose-bleed again.

Of course I was back to one of my old 'theme tunes' – if people would only look for the cause and not just treat the symptoms – it's a song I've been singing for many a year now.

'Which is worse?' I often ask myself, seeing the child distressed, or the worry and sleepless nights the parents endure, hanging on to the edge, looking for an answer that will cure their child.

It was a chilly winter's night and the church bells rang out as I was clearing the snow off my car to go home, when I heard, 'Are you Tony Hogan – the healer?' A tall man approached me, holding a young child in his arms, his wife freezing beside him.

'We've been driving all day from Kerry,' he said. 'But with the snow and trying to find you – we only just got here. Emma is very sick. Can you help us, please?'

I opened the hall door and turned on the lights. Emma lay motionless in his arms, looking pale and withdrawn.

I was concerned when I saw a thick blob of dark olive-green energy around her chest. 'We've never been to Dublin before. Our neighbour told us about you, and gave us directions,' the man said as he lifted Emma's limp body on to my treatment couch. My heart went out to them; they were distressed, cold and exhausted. Emma immediately let out a barking cough and was sick all over me. 'She's been like this for months, getting sick and not sleeping,' said her parents. Emma had chronic asthma. Memories flashed back to my own childhood – when I was unable to breathe or sleep at night with the rattle in my chest, wheezing and vomiting all the time. I gave Emma's parents practical advice I knew would help, but her condition was so bad that I urged them to get her into hospital if she got any worse. 'Emma has been to numerous hospitals already,' they assured me. 'This is the way she is normally.' I calmed down and got to work.

Emma was struggling to breathe, so I concentrated the healing to disperse all the congested blobs of energy trapped around her chest. Soon she started to breathe more easily, the paleness left her cheeks and she even managed a smile. The surprise on her parents' faces told all. 'Oh, it would be a miracle if Emma could sleep, even for one night,' said her mother stroking her poor daughter's head.

I knew they had a long journey back to Kerry, three hundred miles in the snow. So I wasted no time, but asked them to phone me when they arrived home, regardless of the hour. Emma walked down the stairs, hand in hand with her parents, even managing to smile and wave as they set off.

Sure enough, the phone rang at 3.30 in the morning. 'Emma slept all the way home!' said her delighted father, his voice full of hope. His wife came on the phone, thanked me profusely and said it was the first real improvement they'd seen in months.

I was overcome by their happiness, and asked them to phone me later in the day and let me know how Emma was doing. The phone rang that afternoon. It was Emma herself. 'Thank you Mr Hogan for making me better – I'm sorry for being sick all over you,' she said, her voice strong and full of excitement.

Her parents told me she'd slept all through the night. She was hungry when she woke up and wanted a big breakfast. They described all the food she ate. I could hear Emma laughing in the background.

Each week they travelled from Kerry to see me. Emma grew stronger with every visit. I gave her healing to remove the cause – the shock at her birth – and to boost her immune system and strengthen her lungs. I also showed her how to relax and breathe correctly. Then, as the visits became less frequent, she asked if she could take up swimming.

'It would be a great exercise for your lungs,' I encouraged. 'If it's OK with your parents and doctor, then it's perfectly all right with me.'

The family doctor could see the remarkable improvement in the child. He believed in healing, and was both delighted and supportive.

I heard from Emma on and off for a period of time. Then one day, she arrived full of excitement, and asked me to give her strength and confidence for her gala swimming competition. I showed her how to relax and to visualise herself winning. Jokingly I asked her to bring me back a gold and silver medal.

A week later a knock came at the door. Emma stood there, beaming from ear to ear.

'Emma wants to show you something,' announced her parents. Emma stepped forward holding both hands high in the air. Four gold and three silver medals hung from bright red ribbons in her hands. Tears came to my eyes, I felt so proud of her.

Her parents, too, were overwhelmed and gave me a bunch of beautiful flowers and a 'thank you' card.

Children have the biggest and brightest auras of all; bright reds, yellows, orange and green. They're so open-minded and accepting of the healing. Some call me 'The Magic Man'. One little girl asks her mother to 'Take me to the wizard!' whenever she's sick.

Children react quickly to stress and just as quickly get depressed. The three stress areas I look for are – school, home and friends. At home, the more uptight the parents are about their child, the more the child feeds into the cycle of anxiety and fear. So when I'm healing a child, I'm also healing the parents as well.

Two years ago, a beautiful little four-year-old girl named Susan developed a common problem in children called 'constriction of the bowel'. Because of this she was very constipated. Doctors recommended various syrups and tablets, but all to no avail. Her condition got worse.

She became aggravated and tense, and her problem grew into a terrible fear in her young mind. Sometimes she would go to the toilet in her sleep. Her mother takes up the story:

'I was at my wits' end seeing her in such a state, shunting her back and forth to the hospital for tests, feeding her different bottles of medicine and tablets. I thought I was having a nervous break-down. Susan became so upset at our trips to the hospital that both my husband and I felt it was just making her condition worse.

When we first came to see you, I must admit that I was so down in the dumps I was saying to myself, "Here we go again, another dead end." I wasn't hopeful or optimistic at all – I knew if Susan saw another man in a white coat, she'd roar the place down. Well, you didn't wear a white coat and you spoke so kindly to us that Susan sensed this and settled down.

My husband and I were completely gob-smacked at how still and calm she became when you placed your hands on her head and tummy. I've never seen her like this with anyone.

You explained that your healing power reaches the inner

mind and goes directly to the cause. You gently waved your hands over her head to take away her fears.

After that first visit, Susan's condition was totally cured, and she started going to the toilet freely. No fear or panic. I couldn't believe it. And you stopped me having a nervous break-down too! We get on so much better now. I'm so happy that she's well, and we can't thank you enough for making her better.'

It's wonderful when a healing is so obvious that parents and child can see the proof for themselves. A whole new dimension opens between them that didn't exist before.

Moira had just returned from a family holiday to Hong Kong, when her son Neil developed a large cyst on the right side of his face.

It steadily grew in size and turned purple in colour. Neil became embarrassed and self-conscious playing with his pals. Some of his classmates started to taunt him – then the pain began. His mother explained:

'One day Neil came home from school crying. The cyst had begun to pain him terribly and the pain was entering his ear.

The doctor said it was a "sebaceous cyst" – but he could do nothing for it. Neil would have to go to hospital to have it lanced. But the hospital couldn't take him for three weeks and Neil wasn't too keen anyway. By now the pain had got worse. Neil was crying all the time and couldn't sleep at night. A friend suggested I phone you and you came to our house that night. I remember you put your hand on Neil's face, concen-trating on the cyst for some time.

All I can say is that Neil looked so much better and slept all night long, free of pain. When he woke the next morning he took the stairs two at a time, shouting, "It's gone! It's gone!"

The lump, the swelling and that awful purple colour had disappeared. The only evidence left was some blood on his pillow.

Neil sailed into school that morning, delighted with himself, looking ten feet tall. I was so happy for him. No hospital was needed – a miracle had happened!

Neil is now twenty-one and has never had another cyst. We still talk about the night when you gave him healing.

It had a huge effect on Neil. He still talks about it, even to this day.'

Bed-wetting causes so much stress, strain and sleepless nights for all the family. Not only does the child need healing, but also the parents too.

The healing vibrations always flow easily into a child's mind, to where the cause has originated. In the case of Laura she was reacting to her impatient father who disapproved of her behaviour. Her mother said:

'Laura was only four when she developed this dreadful problem of bed-wetting. She would wet the bed several times each night and wake up crying.

We tried everything, even putting nappies on her, but this only made her more upset and angry. Every night she came to our bedroom, distressed and disappointed in herself.

She couldn't bear to be wet. As her problem got worse, she became more hostile to her father, even though we both tried to reassure her, telling her how much we loved her.

These nightly occurrences drained us completely and caused terrible hassle within the family. Our local GP tried different remedies, then recommended we see you.

After the healing, Laura woke the next morning, delighted with herself. She had a completely dry night. "It's just a coincidence," said my husband who was quite sceptical at the time. But night after night her progress continued and he was finally convinced. He even told his friends at work.

Laura is so happy and contented now, it's hard to believe she's the same child.'

Babies have clear, bright auras. Their colours are fine buttercup-yellows, vibrant greens and oranges. Some are transparent, as the baby hasn't developed its thought process and its mind is completely free. Have you ever noticed a baby looking at you? How they look all around you and above your head? This is because they're seeing your aura. This is how they communicate with us.

Our mind aura changes according to our thinking; our emotional aura changes with our feelings. It's at this subtle level where real communication takes place.

When somebody is in deep trouble, they intuitively tune into their spirit companions and ask for help. This sets in motion a chain of events that lead to a solution. A mother's love for a child is an obvious example.

A young woman stood at my door, a baby in her arms. 'I got your name from the taxi driver. I've just come from the hospital – it's my baby, she's bleeding inside. She's dying!' she exclaimed as she grabbed my hand and placed it on her baby's stomach. 'She could die at any moment. Please, could you heal her?' she begged hysterically, gripping my hand tightly.

In an emergency like this, I find myself passing into an altered state of consciousness. Everything starts to spin and I become aware of entering a tunnel, into a spirit dimension, of brilliant white light. I'm aware of many voices around me and I ask for help.

Here on earth, the child's life was in my hands. I felt my body shake inside as the healing energies surged through me, into the baby and her mother. As I was jolted back into the room, I was aware of the mother's hand still holding mine. When I opened my eyes, a beautiful feeling of peace and stillness had filled the room. 'God bless you,' I heard the mother say. Then she left. She hadn't told me her baby's name, or who she was.

But it did not matter, she'd asked God for help and help came to her.

Many years later I was asked to give a talk on healing to a local ladies group. The chairwoman introduced me to seventy women, packed tightly together in a community hall. I began to speak about healing, but soon realised that it was going over their heads. There was an uneasy silence and shuffling of feet. Something prompted me to ask, 'Does anyone here have any experience of healing?'

The chances, I knew, were slim – there were but a handful of healers in the whole of Ireland at the time. The ladies stared at me in blank silence. The chairwoman looked nervous. Suddenly a voice spoke from the back of the hall, 'Excuse me! Excuse me!' Everyone turned towards the woman who was now on her feet.

'You probably don't remember me,' she said. 'But I brought my little baby to see you many years ago – eleven years in fact. I was taking her home from hospital because she was dying. There was no hope. But you put your hands on her and made her better. I heard you were giving this talk tonight – and here she is, my baby. She wants to say something to you.'

A young girl in a red school uniform stood up and made her way through the seats towards me. Looking a bit embarrassed, she blurted out, 'Thanks – thank you.' The atmosphere in the room changed. The women gasped and held their breaths.

Her mother finished telling her story, 'Only for that man there, my little girl wouldn't be here tonight,' she said. The place went wild with clapping and cries of astonishment.

'Yes, I remember you very well,' I said when the chatter subsided. 'I remember you and your little baby. I'm so delighted.' Turning to the crowd I continued, 'Well that's what I do. That's how healing works. I couldn't have said it any better than that.'

The woman joined her daughter and embraced me and gave me flowers. Applause swept through the room. It was a night to remember.

Sometimes I'm asked to help a child who's outside the parameters of healing. My gift, however, means that I never know what will happen until I try.

They'd brought him all the way from Canada. He was seven years old, a young autistic child. I remember he had blue eyes and blond hair and sat looking blankly at the far wall.

His mother – herself a doctor – had booked a hotel for a week so that Stephen could receive healing each day. 'What does she want me to do?' was my first reaction.

'Stephen – Stephen! Look at me. Look at me – look at your mother!' she shouted and clapped her hands vigorously. 'You see – there's no response. Not since he was born, absolutely none!' she said. Stephen's eyes remained in a fixed stare. I waved my hand in front of his face, but there was no reaction. 'My husband is also a doctor and we've had Stephen for every conceivable brain scan and treatment, across Canada and North America – and none of it works for him,' she said despairingly. I pulled up a chair beside them and saw his aura flashing as we talked about him.

Closing my eyes, I placed my hands gently on his forehead and directed healing to his mind, with the intention of opening up the channels in his brain that were shut down. The healing power flowed into him. I felt a door opening in his mind.

His head turned under my hands and I opened my eyes to see him staring up at me. I was stunned when he shouted out, 'Tony! Tony!', and then jumped off the chair to open the door.

We both ran after him to the hall – his mother open-mouthed in amazement – watching as Stephen jumped onto the window ledge, repeating the words, 'Cars – cars!' and pointing to the street below. 'Cars!' he shouted as his mother grabbed his hand and brought him back to the room. 'I can't believe it! I've never heard him speak before,' she kept saying. Both of us were still in shock as Stephen kept naming things that caught his eye.

After healing, Stephen crossed the road with his mother, fully aware of all the cars passing. Before he would just stare ahead in a trance, but now he even responded when the hotel porter play-acted with him. At night he pointed to the sky from his bedroom window, calling out 'Stars – stars' a number of times.

'It was like living with someone who was completely dead,' his mother admitted, all her pent-up anxiety tumbling out. 'My husband and I were at the point of putting him into full-time care. We thought he was lost to us for ever. At last, at last he's come out of that world.'

Children speak the language of the subconscious; they express things in pictures and not in words. Therein lies the secret door to a child's mind. When I first started healing I soon discovered just how truly powerful the mind can be; I began to involve children in their healing and they took to it like a duck to water.

Ben had been in an oxygen tent in the hospital for over three weeks and had to return there. This was the pattern of his life; hospital, home, hospital again. Ben was eleven now and had suffered with chronic asthma all his young life. 'He's spent most of his life in hospital,' his rather sceptical father said when they arrived to see me. 'Nothing can be done for him, except stronger and stronger medication.'

Ben stood beside us gasping for air; he looked as white as a ghost, his chest heaving like a bellows. He was three stone under-weight. When his father left the room, I asked, 'Ben, how would you like to get better for good?' He quickly nodded his approval.

'Well, lie down there on the treatment couch. I'm going to get you to relax and show you how to use your mind, to heal your-self.' His breathing was fast and heavy as he tried to catch air into his lungs.

'I want you to relax your whole body, from head to toe, then travel down into your lungs,' I said, while guiding him through a visualisation exercise. As Ben relaxed more and more I funnelled healing through his energy fields.

Ten minutes passed. I instructed him to 'come back' to the

room – to awaken. Ben opened his eyes and discovered his breathing had magically improved. The pale, ghost-like figure had gone.

His face was bright red, as if he'd been out in the sun for weeks.

Ben smiled as he told me what had happened, his voice now full of fun and magic. 'Well, I travelled down into my lungs, like you said. And saw all these little men dressed in white boiler-suits, going up and down ladders, scrubbing and cleaning all the walls of my lungs.'

'What colour were the walls? I asked.

'They were grey, black and dirty looking. When they had all the walls looking clean, shiny and bright, they began to paint them white. There were hundreds of them, all working together. Up on big ladders and small ladders, and scaffolding.'

I told him how brilliant he was. Effectively he'd triggered his own self-healing power. His visualisation was just perfect.

I called his father in and his astonished look spoke volumes – 'His face looks like a bright red traffic light!' he exclaimed and took Ben back to the hospital. Later he told me the doctors couldn't believe it was the same child. They ran a peak-flow meter test on Ben's lungs – it showed his lung capacity had trebled.

When they sent him home, everyone kept asking where he'd got a suntan from – in the middle of winter! Ben is now in his twenties, married with two children. He's had no further asthmatic attacks.

There are many layers within us that go deeper than the perceived world of thought. Children travel from the heart to the head over time, slowly developing into the conscious world.

When we ask a child what's wrong with them, they can't seem to answer. It isn't any wonder! Children don't function logically – they have a language and a way of perceiving things of their own.

When trying to help a child, I'm never guided by an explanation or theory that went before, or what the parents may have heard. I use all the psychic gifts at my disposal to try and uncover the child's true problem. There are days, however, when I feel like Sherlock Holmes, trying to solve a great mystery.

Alison loved going to school and was the best pupil in her class. Then one day she no longer wanted to go, or to play outside with her friends. She became introverted and afraid. Over a period of a year her parents took her to psychiatrists and psychologists.

Every detail of her life was looked at, all the events leading up to the time when she stopped going to school. No answer was found. She was depressed and they put her on medication. 'It's a complete mystery to us why she's like this,' said her anxious mother. 'We've tried everything. Last week we took her to the zoo and she went hysterical and screamed the place down. We give her a sleeping pill at bedtime, otherwise she won't sleep.'

Alison was eight years old, she didn't want to see another specialist and huddled in the corner of my room, disinterested and fearful. As her mother listed more of her symptoms, I tuned in to her daughter. Alison's aura was barely visible, compressed around her head and shoulders.

I could see shimmering blobs of dark-blue around her head – she had suffered some kind of shock I felt – had lost all faith in her elders and retreated within. There was fear and sadness in her eyes. I decided to take things slowly, not to run at it like a fire-fighter, asking her loads of questions. I knew that others had done this before me. Unbeknown to Alison I directed healing across the room, from my mind to hers and watched as her aura brightened. She responded instantly to my healing.

When Alison came again, I gave her a sheet of paper and some crayons and asked her to draw me a picture.

'What will I draw?' she asked playfully, no longer feeling under scrutiny. 'Draw me a tree,' I replied and set about answering my absent healing letters. In a situation like this, I need the patience and co-operation of the parents.

It's not always forthcoming, 'When will she be better – when do you think she'll be back in school – how long will it take?' I'm asked frequently. This puts pressure on me and the person I'm trying to help.

Alison's parents were no different; each visit the questions kept coming. Yet, week after week, Alison became more settled in herself and looked forward to our meetings. Finally, all the hard work and patience paid off. Alison took out her sketch pad one day, and drew a fish with great big teeth.

'What's that?' I asked.

'It's a piranha fish,' she replied. Her aura I could see was flashing around her, expanding and shrinking. It meant she was reacting to shock or trauma. I knew instantly I was on to a winner.

'They eat big people and little children,' Alison said.

'Where did you see them?'

'At school – it was on the film.'

Bingo! There was the answer. Alison had seen a film in school about 'man-eating piranha fish' and it was there her fear developed. Her parents and teacher confirmed she had seen the film. She was terrified of going to school after that.

When the TV was on, she wouldn't look at it in case she saw the piranha. She screamed in the zoo because she was in the aquarium, being shown the fish. This intense fear had played on her young mind. I asked Alison if she'd like to get rid of that monster fish for good. 'Yes' she shouted. I got her to relax and close her eyes and to imagine a dolphin. 'Flipper! I can see Flipper the dolphin,' she said.

'Great – now Flipper is going to help you. See yourself swimming with Flipper.'

She began to laugh. 'The piranha is way in the distance.'

'Now I want you to see Flipper swim towards the piranha fish – see him eat the piranha fish!' There was silence for a moment. 'Yippee!' she shouted, 'Flipper ate him all up – now he's tickling me,' she giggled.

'Anytime you're afraid Alison, you can close your eyes and see your friend Flipper. He will help you,' I said finally. Alison went back to school and played with her friends. She had no more depression or fear and no more sleepless nights.

Some children are born very sensitive and are often quite psychic. Their parents either accept they've a gifted child, or create fear and upset around the child.

I've seen many children under medication attending psychiatrists because no one saw their natural gift.

I recognised Brian's grandmother immediately. She'd been to see me years earlier with a frozen shoulder and arthritis in her spine and knees.

'You did a great job on me Mr Hogan. I've never had as much as a pain or an ache since. I'm eighty this year,' she said with a smile. Her daughter and grandson sat with her in the waiting room. 'Can I have a wee word with you first?' she asked, and slipped into my healing room, closing the door behind her.

'Come here 'til I tell you – it's about wee Brian outside. I don't want my daughter to hear what I'm going to tell you.' I moved my chair closer to hear her whispering. 'Brian's only nine, but he has a little friend – you know, an invisible friend.

'He talks to him all day long and his mother and father don't understand. They think he's mad. They brought him to three, you know, … those people in white coats?'

'Psychiatrists?' I suggested.

'Yes! – those fellows. They have Brian doped up to the eyeballs, the poor lad. He loves coming to stay with me and tells me all about his little pal, but his parents don't understand. His father can't take it any more and wants him put away. Get rid of the problem – lock him up.

'I was at my wits' end and thought to myself – who could help the poor wee fellow? Immediately you came into my mind. You're the only one who understands. You're psychic, Tony. I knew the very first day I met you. You have the gift.'

I nodded in agreement. She reminded me so much of my own grandmother. 'I'll send Brian in and keep his mother outside for a while. She doesn't understand what you do,' she said.

Brian came in and sat up on a stool. I could feel the intense fear coming off him – from the threat of being put away by his parents.

'Your grandmother is a lovely woman,' I began. 'She tells me you've a friend. What's his name?' There was a long pause. Brian struggled for his voice.

'Peter,' he whispered.

'He's a lot younger than yourself?'

'He's – kinda five.'

'What's he doing walking around the room?'

Brian turned to look at his friend, then hung his head for a moment. Very slowly he looked up at me and asked, 'Can you see him?'

'Of course I can. He's looking out the far window.'

Brian glanced around.

'When you came into the room, Peter stood on your left side. Then he began to skip across the room,' I said.

Brian's face lit up.

'You really can see him?'

'Of course I can. I had invisible friends too when I was young – and I still have them. They help me all the time in my healing work. It's just that some adults don't see them and it makes them afraid.'

'What can I do? I'm upsetting my Mum and Dad. They're going to lock me up!' he said, shaking.

I tuned in to my spirit friends and the solution gushed through.

'Brian, there's nothing wrong with you – you're perfectly normal. You've a wonderful gift, it's just that your parents don't appreciate it. It's not their fault. Some adults don't understand what I'm doing either. But like you, I had a very caring grandmother who understood me.'

Brian was silent for a moment, taking it all in.

'How would you feel, if you were to leave your friend Peter with me?' I said.

'I'll look after him, and any time you wish you can see him again. Just ask your grandmother to bring you back here and I'll reawaken your gift.'

'You mean I'll be normal and my Mum and Dad won't be angry any more?'

'No, your Mum and Dad won't be angry any more,' I reassured him.

Brian was so delighted, he agreed and I gave him healing. Before he left, he waved a final goodbye to his friend Peter. And when we opened the door, his mother had her ear pressed up to it and blurted out, 'Doctor! Will he end up in a nut-house? Is he gone mad? My husband is upset with him talking to himself!'

I stopped her short and assured her that Brian was fine and a very intelligent child. Brian's grandmother gave him a big hug and reiterated, 'Yes! He's such an intelligent lad.'

'Brian never looked back after seeing you, Tony,' she said on the phone to me three months later.

'His parents are delighted, especially his father. There's no mention of those people in white coats any more. He's off the tablets and out playing with his friends. He's so happy.' Then she became serious for a moment.

'Brian told me everything you said to him, Tony – about his little friend and that. And I was wondering would it affect him in any way – not having the gift?'

'Not at all,' I said. 'His gift is there within him. All he needs to do is tap into it, any time he wishes.'

EXERCISE – HEALING FOR YOUR CHILD

Here is a wonderful healing exercise I've recommended to parents over the years, and I share it with you.

Place your hand on your child's head, before they go off to sleep at night. Gently stroke the child's head as if rubbing away all fears and anxieties from the mind.

Speak softly the following words of encouragement – whatever you feel is appropriate for your child:

❧ You're having more confidence in yourself.
❧ You're making more friends in school.
❧ You're breathing more easily.
❧ You're enjoying your maths/English/history.
❧ You're getting on better with your teacher.
❧ You're more secure in yourself.
❧ You're getting on better with your brother/sister.
❧ You're expressing yourself much better.
❧ You're enjoying your swimming/running/hockey/tennis.

Now gently stroke their forehead a few times and repeat slowly the following words, 'Sleep … Sleep … Sleep.' If you wish to add any further positive words please do so. Do this every night for six weeks and see your child change for the better.

CHAPTER 7

THEY SUFFERED IN SILENCE

'A mighty flame followeth a tiny spark.'

Dante

THE PERSON WHO HAS HAD the greatest influence on my work as a healer is a man called Harry Edwards. He was born in England on 29 May 1893 and devoted his whole life to healing. Famous for his public demonstrations, some of my patients would travel by boat and train to see the great healer in action in London's Royal Albert Hall. Before an audience of thousands, Harry Edwards demonstrated his remarkable gift of healing – very often healing the sick and the incurable.

My patients told him of my healing work, which delighted him greatly; he spoke of the struggle that lay ahead of me, working on my own in Ireland, and regularly sent his best wishes through the Irish people who came to him for healing.

I wasn't a 'faith healer' or 'a seventh son of a seventh son', who

– as folklore would have it – could heal traditional ailments. I knew that Harry Edwards called his work 'spirit healing' or 'spiritual healing', but what was I?

Through much soul-searching and spiritual guidance from my spirit friends, it became clear to me that I was indeed a spiritual healer – just like Harry Edwards.

As I travelled the length and breadth of Ireland, however, I found that the term 'spiritual healing' wasn't acceptable to some – they were more comfortable with the old labels.

Harry Edwards passed away in 1976, and although I never shook his hand our paths crossed time and time again.

Alice's first healing experience was at the hands of Harry Edwards, before she came to see me:

'As a young child I always had this strange feeling that the world was tumbling down around me. I was experiencing terrible fears and panic attacks but didn't realise it then. As I grew up, these fears steadily became worse; I experienced sheer terror of travelling, of heights, walking up a hill was just too much for me. Being asked to go to the shops would send me into a blind panic. The worst fear of all was the fear of dying, which would engulf me every day. I never told anyone how I was feeling, not even my best friends.

As I went through my teenage years I became more and more dependent on trusted friends. In my twenties I developed a severe back. A good friend told me that she was going over to England to see a spiritual healer and would I like to come. Without thinking about it too much, I got the courage from somewhere, and we took the ferry boat and train.

A coach met us at the station and took us to Mr Edwards's house in Burrows Lea, outside the town of Guildford in Surrey.

I didn't know what to expect when we arrived. There were three healers on that day: Olive Burton, Ray Branch and

Harry Edwards. People had come from all over the world for healing. Harry Edwards called me over. He had a lovely caring smile and snow-white hair; I immediately felt at peace with him. 'What can I do for you?' he asked.' I told him about the problem with my back and of my lifelong fears and phobias. He looked at me with a wide smile and put his great big hand on my back. The pain just went away; the relief was instant. I couldn't believe it.

Mr Edwards talked about my phobias and said he would help me cope with them through his absent healing intercessions, which he promised to do every day. I kept in touch by letter with Mr Edwards and over time I began to feel more confident within myself. Then one day his secretary wrote to tell me that Mr Edwards had passed away. I was devastated by the news; Mr Edwards had been a beacon of light that suddenly went out of my life.

Over months my fears and phobias became more pronounced again. My doctor put me on strong medication but that didn't help. I remember sitting in the doctor's waiting room, when I got a severe panic attack, and thought the walls were coming in on top of me. Then I felt everyone was looking at me. After that I never returned. I simply couldn't.

As time went on I became a prisoner in my own home. The outside world didn't exist for me any more. My friends would call for me every day, but I had to keep making excuses about why I couldn't go out. Eventually the doorbell stopped ringing. I had lost all my friends. I suppose they became sick of me being sick. The downstairs living room became too big for me so I had to retreat to my bedroom to feel safe. I lived there for twelve long years on my own, my days spent crying, hunched in a corner — my body trembling and shaking all over. Death was the only answer that was left; the only escape route I had open to me. At night while trying to sleep I would experience a big lump in my throat that prevented me from breathing. To stop breathing would send me into a terrible state of panic. I would end up kicking and screaming on the floor, trying to catch my breath back. That's how I struggled to live all those years.

One morning my father was in the front garden clipping the hedge, when he began to chat to our neighbour Joan, who was passing. He told her about the state I was in and asked if she was passing again would she be kind enough to look in on me for a chat. There and then, Joan came up the stairs to my bedroom. We chatted for a while and she told me that she too had the same problem a year before and was helped by a spiritual healer. She asked me would I like to meet him.

'How can I travel to England when I haven't been outside the house for over twelve years?' I asked. Joan explained that you weren't that far away.

My heart lifted as I immediately thought of Harry Edwards and the help he gave me all those years ago. Joan brought me to you in a taxi. When I walked into your healing room, there hanging on the wall right behind you was a picture of Harry Edwards! I couldn't believe it. It was as if Mr Edwards himself had led me to you.

You knew straight away how I was feeling and what I was going through. I was stunned when you told me about the choking episodes and how you understood my fears and phobias. You said in order for healing to be effective and lasting you needed to heal the deeper cause. It would take time for the rays of healing power to restore my body, mind and spirit back to full health. It was fine with me; I didn't care how long it took!

You asked me to relax in the chair and close my eyes. A tremendous amount of heat came from your hands. Gradually all the stress and tension of twelve long years began running out from my body like a river; it was a magical sensation. When you placed your hands on my head, I could feel this incredible peace and stillness envelop me. I felt as if I were wrapped in a blanket of heavenly peace. All that day I remember my feet weren't walking on the ground, but floating above it. It was an incredible feeling – I suppose I was walking on air.

Two visits later I was able to do my own shopping. Eventually I ventured into town – another miracle. There were physical benefits too; I had had a continuous sinus problem for years, which cleared. I had also had what the doctor called a large goitre swelling on my neck for years, and this went away gradually. Behind my ears I had a cluster of little cysts. I asked you to put your healing hands on them and the following morning, while brushing my hair, I discovered to my amazement that they had all disappeared. You explained that all these physical problems were manifestations of my mental state.

I remember, during healing, having flashbacks of memories of the past, things I had completely forgotten about. While sitting in the waiting room I would say to myself, "I'm not going to tell Tony about them." I would block out all my negative thoughts but once I sat down on the chair, every single thought I was thinking came pouring out.

You explained that there were different stages to my recovery, that you were healing all my past memories – all the baggage I had been carrying around inside. On my final visit, much to my surprise, I had the most beautiful spiritual experience of my entire life. No sooner had you placed your hands on my head and I closed my eyes when I saw an incredible rainbow with coloured streams of light pouring through me. This experience seemed to go on forever. From that moment I knew I was completely healed.'

There are some people who suffer with mental illness that is more difficult to treat, especially if they are not in control of their own minds.

It was coming up to lunch-time and there was only one more person to see. 'Next please,' I called into the waiting room and walking back into my healing room, I turned to see a young woman in a most magnificent white lace wedding dress with jewellery to match, looking at me.

'Please, sit down.' I said. 'Is it your first time to come for healing?'

'Yes,' she said. Putting on her white veil she began to fluff it out.

'It's not very often I get a bride coming to see me on her wedding day.' I said. She just smiled.

'When is the wedding?' I continued.

'Three-thirty.' She spoke in a soft country accent.

'I better hurry up so,' I replied glancing up at the clock on the wall.

Her name was Diana and she worked as a hairdresser. I took down some details about her health and medical history. She told me she had suffered from depression for years. Sure enough her aura registered the usual dark heavy clouds I was used to seeing.

'Who's the lucky man?' I asked.

There was a stony silence. Her head lowered. After a moment she raised her head and looked through her veil straight at me in the eye and said 'You ...!'

I got a shock but composed myself. It was then I noticed her wedding ring.

'Have you been married before?' I asked nervously.

'Yes,' she replied firmly, 'I'm married to Peter, but today I'm marrying you!'

I quickly thought to myself, I won't be getting married today because I've got a poor man suffering with cancer coming up on the train from Wexford at half-past-three!

Eventually I talked the woman into letting me telephone her husband Peter, who came along and collected her.

In my clinic and in psychiatric hospitals, I've observed those who are mentally disturbed. The most common trait in all of these sufferers is a constant rocking back-and-forth motion of the body. Over the years I've wondered why this pattern is so prevalent in mentally disturbed patients and so I began using my psychic gifts to see what was happening in their aura. I discovered that the sufferer's electrical energy field was overcharged, and as a result the rocking motion was a natural process. It enabled the person to disperse the build-up of energy out of the body.

With most of my work I find I am boosting people's energy levels, but with mentally disturbed people and those who are elated I do the opposite. I stabilise them by dispersing or scattering their over-charged energy field, thereby taking pressure off their nervous system.

People who are 'unstable' are often over-sensitive to their surroundings. They are 'thin-skinned' and lack the necessary skills to function in their everyday lives. Their energy fields are often thin and wispy. They lack 'presence' and self-confidence, and hide from people for fear of being hurt.

Healing is marvellous in strengthening self-confidence and freeing people to live positive lives, doing the things they want to do, instead of living lives of complete misery.

Many depressed people are emotionally blocked, out of touch with their true feelings. If I ask them how they feel about something, a look of surprise passes across their face as they struggle for an answer.

I asked one man recently how he felt about the loss of his wife. 'You'll have to ask my doctor about that,' was his reply. It's an answer I've heard all too frequently over the years.

People who are frequently sick have never been asked how they feel; no connection is made between the two. I firmly believe if we don't care for the emotional side of our nature, the physical body will eventually fall ill.

Someone who is open, in touch with their feelings, is far easier to heal than the person who's blocking them out. Children, for example, tend to be far easier to heal than adults, simply because they've not learnt how to suppress their feelings.

We all have our own unique wisdom from spirit; and through the doorway of our feelings we access our higher intuition to enable us to solve life's problems.

I have sometimes gone out on a limb to interpret a feeling and show it to the patient. This feeling was 'screaming' to be heard. Sadly, however, some don't want to hear this advice.

'So you're the great healer Tony Hogan,' he roared. Gus was his name. You could tell by his loud, brash voice he was used to giving orders. He announced he was a sergeant in the army and thought I was going to stand up and salute him.

I took one look at his fragmented aura and replied, 'Are you an alcoholic?' Visibly stunned, he stopped dead in his tracks. I could hear my invisible friends say, 'We have a right one here!'

'How long have you been an alcoholic?' I continued.

'I've drank most of my army life. But I've changed for the sake of my niece Pauline who's outside,' he barked. 'She's the one brought me here, to see you. Her aunt died a while ago and left her £30,000. If I come to see you and stay off the drink, she'll buy me a taxi-plate,' he boasted.

'This guy is going to drink every penny of it.' I could hear my spirit friends say.

I took one look at him and asked, 'Is that the truth?'

His face turned red with anger; I told him that healing would- n't work on someone who was dishonest. I asked him to leave. He called for Pauline and slammed the door on his way out. I ran to the top of the stairs and asked Pauline to come back, as I wanted to give her a message. Her uncle stood fuming as she came back up the stairs. I ushered her into my room and as I closed the door I could feel the strong presence of her aunt around her.

'Pauline,' I said. 'Your uncle is going to drink every penny of your aunt's money. That's the message I'm being asked to pass on to you.'

She looked at me with complete surprise and said, 'No, he won't. He gave me his word he won't ever take a drink again, and I believe him. He's been so good to me in the past few weeks.'

One year later, a letter arrived from Pauline. 'I'm so ashamed to tell you that my uncle drank it all, every penny of it. He eventually tricked me into giving him all the money, the whole £30,000. Why, why didn't I listen to you that day?'

Some people aren't ready to appreciate the supreme efforts that spirit is making in trying to help them. A woman in her forties with a goitre problem sat opposite me. I knew from the moment she entered the room she wasn't a suitable candidate for healing.

'How can I help you?' I asked, knowing full well she was only here because of a well-meaning friend, waiting outside.

She told me her name was Noreen, removed a bright orange silk scarf from around her neck and showed me her throat. 'As you can see, it's my throat. They tell me it's a goitre.' I moved closer to have a look.

'I have seen far bigger goitre conditions,' I said. 'How is it bothering you?'

She looked sharply at me and said, 'I throw a lot of dinner parties. I can't wear a low-cut dress any more.'

'Does it affect you in any other way?' I enquired.

'Not really – no. My man [her specialist] told me to come in any time and he'll just whip it out.'

'I see,' I said. 'Well as regards healing, I can't promise you anything. It could take a while to sort it out, and you'd have to come for a few sessions. Is that all right with you?'

'But my man could have it out in the morning!' she retorted.

I was getting the message loud and clear – I wasn't her man.

'Did your man tell you if there were side effects to the operation?' I asked finally.

'Heavens no. My man just said to come in any time and he'll whip it out!' she insisted. 'I've made up my mind right now. I'll ring him first thing Monday morning and have it removed.'

Two years passed. The friend who brought her came to see me one day with one of her children. 'How did everything work out with your friend with the goitre problem?' I asked.

'She's been house-bound ever since she had the operation. Everything went terribly wrong Tony, she's on so many tablets, you wouldn't recognise her. I drop down to see her most days and all she keeps saying to me is, "Why didn't I listen to that man?"'

Sceptics have compressed auras that reflect a narrow mind and outlook. They lack the range or frequency to look beyond their limited way of thinking; nothing is allowed in or out.

An eminent scientist came to see me one day for healing. I took one look at his mind aura and could see it was very tight and shallow around his head. So I decided to restrict my explanation on how healing works and just gave him a brief outline. When I had finished, he looked up and asked, 'Is your healing something to do with trees …?'

Frequently I meet people who are struggling with their illness, without any encouragement or support, sometimes even from their own families. This puts further pressure on me, as I have to support them emotionally too.

I had been healing people up and down the country for many years when there was an upsurge in religious prayer healing; people were told not to go to anyone 'outside the pale' as it were.

Angela had a hard life bringing up four children, having lost her husband to cancer and her only other support system, her mother. She lived a life of humble devotion to the church. Every day she cleaned the church and kept appointments.

Then one day hospital tests showed she had cancer of the throat and oesophagus. Her whole world fell apart. As a regular member of the local prayer group, she had various priests and nuns pray over her.

She slipped into a deep depression at the thought of leaving her four young children behind, since they would most likely be put into a home. Angela struggled to carry out her duties in the church and visiting some sick people from her community in hospital. One day she got engaged in a conversation with one of the nurses who suggested that she come to see me for healing.

I could tell straight away she was a very humble person and she responded instantly to my healing. On the first visit her depression lifted and all the upset in her life came tumbling out. Over a couple of months the inflammation in her chest and throat eased, her appetite returned and she put weight back on. She continued to receive healing. One day she came to see me and said, 'I believe the cancer's gone.'

I suggested that she have it checked out in the hospital. A week later Angela returned to confirm that indeed the cancer was no longer there.

'They asked me in the hospital what I had done with myself. I told them I went to you for healing and as I was leaving they said, I was a very lucky woman.'

I was so delighted for Angela. She was somebody who really deserved a second chance. She gave me a great big hug and lifted me right off the ground, she was so delighted with herself. A few weeks later she returned looking very down. 'What's the matter?' I asked.

'I went home and told everyone about the incredible results from your healing. When word got round in the community and the parish priest found out he was livid. I've been stopped from helping out in the church, and banned from attending the prayer group.' Tears flowed down her face. 'I really miss it Tony. I feel so upset inside.'

She calmed down and continued, 'It's the parish priest, he said unless you write him a letter saying that he was the one that healed my cancer, and not you, he won't allow me back to the church.'

'I can't understand this Angela. You have been healed of cancer. Is he not delighted that you are better?' I said.

'He doesn't see it that way. He wants you to write him a letter saying it wasn't you that healed me,' she said.

I couldn't believe what I was hearing, it was like something out of the Dark Ages. I turned to Angela and said, 'I cannot deny the healing gift that I have been given. I'm sorry I cannot write such a letter.'

I tuned in to my spirit friends for a solution. 'Tell him it was God that healed you.' Before I had finished my sentence, she said, 'He wouldn't accept that either, it must be a personal letter from you.'

At that point I got really mad. 'Surely he knows it doesn't matter who the instrument was that healed you, the most important thing is you have been healed?' Angela sobbed her heart out, she could see no way through her dilemma.

When she had finished crying I looked Angela straight in the eye and spoke from the heart, 'You and your children have to live in the community for the rest of your lives. The main thing is you are healthy again, your whole life is ahead of you and what's important is your welfare. Tell your priest you won't be coming to see me again, tell him I said it was God who healed you and not me.' I never saw Angela again.

Shock and trauma go to the very core of our inner being. They are absorbed in the deepest part of us, our spirit, and register on the energy counterpart of our physical body. Taking the shock and trauma out of a person's spirit can be likened to taking a splinter out of the skin. People have turned to me over the years because nobody could see the splinter. Bandage over bandage covered the wound, but the wound still festered deep within the person's being.

Many people come to see me in states of complete hopelessness and despair due to some kind of personal experience they have had in their lives. Some told me of their horror of hospital and the awful treatment they received. For others, it was the abuse they'd suffered in their formative years in school. Many people from the war in Northern Ireland had seen members of their family murdered. Others lived through the bombing and gunfire, experiencing death all around them. Over the years I sat and listened to many stories of heartache and pain.

Some came from numerous wars around the world: from Africa, Romania, South America, Angola, the former Yugoslavia, Iran, Iraq and the Philippines.

'One day everything was normal,' Jasmine told me, while crying her eyes out. She had come from Kuwait, and was suffering with severe shock and depression.

'The next day the Iraqi soldiers poured on to the streets, the noise of bombs going off and rifle fire just terrifying us.'

She hid for months in a sealed basement fearing for her life, only coming up at night for water and food, sneaking out of the hole and sneaking back in again. Her husband hid there permanently terrified of being shot, or imprisoned by the Iraqi army. She coped as best she could. It was a never-ending nightmare, she told me, hearing the gunfire and screaming, wondering who was being killed.

The shock and trauma of the Gulf War was all too much for her. When it was finally over, her nightmare continued. Her nerves were shattered, her life was over, she couldn't cope with living. Depression set in, followed by a complete nervous breakdown. Then Jasmine heard about me from an Irish nurse who worked in the main hospital where she was a patient.

After only one session of hands-on healing Jasmine wrote a letter to me from Kuwait, saying that that day in my healing room the dreadful war had ended.

Georgina, a young woman from Greece, sat in her bed in the psychiatric hospital in Dublin terrified out of her wits. She was twenty-four when she had her first baby, but soon after she developed postnatal depression and was committed to hospital. While on strong anti-depressants her mind became distorted. Figures came out of the television and raced towards her. Rats and mice ran up and down the wall; everyone took on a sinister look. She cried all day in bed, terrified, the blankets over her head.

'Now Georgina,' the doctor said, 'On Monday morning we are taking you down for shock treatment – to help you.'

That news was the straw that finally broke the camel's back. Georgina was in despair and all alone. Beneath the blankets she cried out for help, asking God for mercy. Footsteps came and went. She heard a voice saying, 'Well, how are you today?'

The woman in the bed beside her had a visitor. Georgina listened to the conversation while under the blankets.

At the mention of my name and the words 'spiritual healing', she piped up immediately, asking the woman for my name and telephone number. Georgina clung on to that piece of paper like a piece of gold until her husband arrived from work.

'Will you telephone this man? Ask him can I see him. Tell him it's urgent, please hurry,' she urged.

The next evening Georgina arrived at my clinic with her husband. She told of her horror at the prospects of facing shock treatment. I could immediately see the trauma embedded in her.

I gave her healing and when she returned three days later she looked radiant. Her husband couldn't stop shaking my hand. I was delighted for them both. A few months passed and a beautiful thank-you card arrived in the post with a happy family photograph of the two of them with their young baby.

A common experience shared by many is the loss of a loved one. Grief isn't an illness. There's no surgery or tablet that will cure it. The person's secure world is broken into little pieces. The shock and trauma of the loss is felt at the core of the person's being. Some struggle through their days in a state of numbness. Others are so traumatised and heartbroken that their spirit temporarily removes itself from the physical body; they are 'beside themselves' with grief.

Intense anger is just one of many emotions felt; there is a desire to blame someone else for the loss or even the deceased person. A common response of the grieving person is, 'Why did he leave me, why did he not say goodbye?'

Another important factor is how the death occurred. An unexpected death in a car crash, falling off a building or drowning creates a sudden shock, which is followed by numbness, denial and disbelief. Those who are bereaved replay the event over and over in an attempt to come to terms with what's happened.

When death is the result of a murder, the feeling is of intense anger and a need to take revenge. These forms of grief can take a long time to work through.

There is also the death of a loved one due to suicide, which invokes an overwhelming feeling of powerlessness. The bereaved blame themselves for being unable to prevent the suicide. In order to heal, people need to work through their grief, allowing themselves to acknowledge all of their feelings. There are those who are completely loyal, afraid to tell you how they really feel, in case they are letting a loved one down in some way, yet when a person acknowledges their true feelings about life as it was, very often this is the turning point in the grieving process.

The death of an animal can be equally traumatic. An elderly person living on their own with a dog or a cat can view the pet as a faithful friend and companion, with which they have shared a whole lifetime of experiences.

Apart from feeling bereaved they also feel completely isolated; no one takes them seriously and a remark such as 'It's only an animal' can compound the pain and grief felt.

People who come for healing suffering with suppressed grief, buried from somewhere in their past may not have grieved properly for a parent or loved one. This manifests itself in many different forms: bouts of fear or panic attacks, extreme possessiveness of a child or partner, sleeplessness, intense feelings of insecurity and bouts of crying for no apparent reason. Suppressed grief can often be triggered at the birth of a child. It highlights the absence of a loved one, for example a parent.

Because of the unique insight and experience that I have about life and death, I am able to give understanding, inner peace and comfort to help the bereaved move through their grief and carry on with their lives.

Colette came to see me suffering with depression as a direct result of losing her father. This is her experience:

'I never had brothers or sisters. My mother passed away many years ago. So I was left to look after my father whom I nursed for several years, making sure he had everything he needed. I can honestly say I lived for him because I loved him very much. We had a great relationship. My only outlets were my work and my father and, when he died, part of me died with him. I sunk into a deep depression and lost all confidence.

Every night I would just sit in the house all on my own weeping. It always showed on my face the next day in work, which made me very embarrassed. One of the girls dropped your card on my desk. I kept it in my bag until one day I felt completely distraught and I telephoned to make an appointment.

I remember that very first evening, while waiting for the bus, I turned back many times to go home. I felt completely hopeless and lost. Then a strange feeling of peace came over me, I felt my father urging me to go on.

When I arrived at your place I felt I had come home. You listened, you understood, you filled in the missing pieces about death and what happens.*

I now feel even closer to my father than I ever did before. I

---

* For more on this see Chapter 13

133

have so many friends and so much to do with my life. You made
a new woman out of me.'

Mary was thirty-one years of age, working in a government depart-
ment. She came to see me after the second miscarriage in less than
a year. This is her story:

'My first miscarriage was an early one and within the space of
twenty-seven weeks I conceived again. I was admitted to hospi-
tal bleeding and in dreadful pain.
*   The bottom of my world fell out as we buried our baby, Alan.*
*   When I first started going to see you, Tony, I had written you*
a letter one night. I was on my own and felt quite suicidal. I
felt that nobody could help me. In the letter I stated I had noth-
ing but health problems. I was quite overweight and bloated all
the time. I had high blood pressure, coeliac disease, a dreadful
skin rash all over my body [eczema] and I was a heavy smoker.
I felt very down, lacking in confidence and quite depressed.'

I remember Mary coming to see me that morning. She sat across
from me with her head down. She couldn't speak for fear of falling
apart but handed me the letter outlining her problems. At the end
of it she wrote, 'Please, please help me. I need help badly!' As I read
the letter I tuned in to Mary and felt her deep sorrow.

She was starting out early in her married life, yet everything
seemed to be going wrong for her and her husband; they had been
married a couple of years and would have loved to start a family. Her
story continues:

'When you finished reading the letter, I asked you when could I
have a baby. You were very nice and kind, and said, 'We'll take
one step at a time.' You placed your hands on the back of my neck.
*   I don't know how you knew I was in pain there. I had a*

terrible headache at the time. All I know is when I left your clinic the pain was gone. On the way out the door I felt so good, the relief was instant. It was as though I had let out a deep sigh 'Phew!' and felt help was on the way.

That day I went home and slept very well, something I hadn't done in years. The next morning I felt I had loosened up inside and began to sail through life. I became more relaxed and happier in myself.

The depression had been lifted and I became more in touch with the happy side of myself, which I thought that I had lost for ever. Then, within three weeks of going for healing, my blood pressure went down. All the bloatedness in my body disappeared. The skin rash that plagued me for five years vanished.

Within two months I was pregnant again. You helped me to give up smoking – a major step forward as I had been addicted. I looked great and felt great. The whole pregnancy was bliss.

I had a beautiful baby girl, Laura. I was over the moon.

A few years later, against all the odds, I had a lovely baby boy. We called him Nicholas.'

When a person who is sick, outside the reach of medical science, and classed as incurable, begins to show signs of getting better, some people are fearful and suspicious. Instead of being happy for them they almost disapprove.

I remember one man coming to see me with an incurable condition. After healing he began to outlive his time; by rights he should have been dead by now, according to the doctors. 'People keep asking why I'm still walking around and looking so well,' he said apologetically. When the first year passed he told me he felt he had to keep apologising to everyone. As the second year flew by he really began to get worried. The pressure came on him.

The third year he stayed in his house, he felt so embarrassed for living so long!

Is it any wonder that when some people get better, they keep the good news to themselves?

Betty had stomach cancer. She told me her sister Maureen (whom she hadn't seen in years) gave her instructions to rush home after seeing me so that she could pick out the dress and jewellery she was to be buried in. Betty's anger kept welling up inside.

When the healing session was over, Betty stood up and said, 'That sister of mine has another thing coming if she thinks I'm going to die on the time and day that she demands. After this, Tony, I'm going into town shopping!'

When people with very serious complaints come to see me, they invariably bring with them their medical history – typed up and full of detail. While it helps to give me a picture of where the person is coming from, the information in itself is of little use; it only reveals the numerous dead-ends the person has been down in trying to find a cure.

It is, however a point of reference from which to begin healing. Any improvement from then on is a miracle in itself.

Kate came with a large, bulging medical file tucked under her arm. This is her horrendous and remarkable story:

'My nightmare began fifteen years ago. I experienced severe pain in my right side and was rushed by ambulance to the nearest hospital. The doctors, thinking it was a kidney problem, carried out numerous tests and released me soon after. Some time later, however, I collapsed and was rushed back to hospital, this time for emergency surgery. They removed an ovarian cyst and I left three weeks later, unable to straighten up, with the same terrible pain gripping my side. I continued attending the hospital and was put on medication. Six months after the first operation, they discovered I had endometriosis, a problem with the lining of the womb. My own doctor carried out the second operation, to remove adhesions and clean up the endometriosis, which had spread so rapidly.

I struggled on for another three-and-a-half years, under medication, going back and forth to the hospital. The side-effects were awful – nausea, headaches, acute pains in my back arms and legs; tiredness, bloatedness, terrible depression. Eventually I changed hospitals. My new doctor said I had a large lump on my ovary and would need a hysterectomy.

He also told me that I had only one ovary left – the first doctor must have taken out the other when he removed the cyst. I had the hysterectomy and was fine for six months, but slipped back to square one again. The pain and nausea were acute. I was sick all day long, very tired, with a dragging feeling in my side that went into my lower stomach. The hospital put me on stronger drugs but the side-effects were even worse. I couldn't sleep. I was uptight and disinterested in everything. I became totally depressed. My doctor didn't know what to do with me. I struggled on for another year until I collapsed at home one evening.

My doctor was away on holiday and I was in severe pain so they rushed me to another hospital. I tried to tell them of my medical history, but they went ahead anyway and removed my appendix. Two weeks later I was home again with the same intense pain. On returning from his holidays, my doctor blew a fuse when he heard they'd removed my appendix. He ran more tests, but held out little hope that any further treatment would be successful. At this point I'd given up; the future looked black with no light at the end of the tunnel. I was once an outgoing person, but now I was little more than an invalid. I really felt I would end up in a mental hospital. I ate painkillers like Smarties and went around like a zombie. Time passed in a fog and I ended up in hospital again. I was referred to yet another doctor – a general surgeon who ran his own clinic. He said it was a recurrence of the endometriosis and not a new problem. They operated again and I was sent home on heavy medication. I had lost so much weight by now that everyone thought I was dying.

November 1987 came and I awoke with an intense pain in my chest. I thought I was having a heart attack. Again I was rushed into hospital and put on a drip.

They ran numerous tests and did scans of my kidneys, which showed up two large cysts on either side. These, I was told, had been causing the pain all along. I had major surgery to remove both cysts – apparently they'd grown into my bowel. Two weeks later I was released from hospital and sent home in dreadful pain.

Over the years I'd spent a fortune on doctors, going back and forth to the hospital every other day, but the pain was still there. I was totally cheesed off with the doctors and felt miserable, with no hope for the future. My friend Susan saw me going from bad to worse. One morning I said to her, "I can't take this any more."

"Would you not try something else?" she asked.

"Like what?"

"Would you not try spiritual healing?"

"I can't see that helping me," I snapped.

Susan had been very good to me, so reluctantly I made an appointment to see you. I was really very sceptical. Healing was for someone else, I thought, and would be of no benefit to me. The morning I came to see you, I was at the end of my tether doubled up in pain, feeling like an old woman. I told you of my history. You placed your hands on my tummy, and on my back and head. When I came away that morning, I felt that a great big cloud had lifted – all the pain left me. My head was completely clear and I felt really good. Susan noticed the change straight away – "I told you Tony would make you better," she said. Rather reluctantly I replied, "Well, maybe." The pain came back the following day but this time it wasn't *as bad. It was as if I'd stepped out of the pain. I felt an inner strength.*

The painkillers used to stop the pain for a short time, but left me feeling sick and muzzy. This was a miracle! I remember I had no pain that first weekend and ate everything around me.

For the very first time I was able to cope. A few weeks later I felt so well, that I went dancing 'til four in the morning. The pain came and went, but there were more good days than bad days, and in a matter of weeks, the pain vanished completely.

I went on holiday to France and it was the best holiday I'd ever been on – off medication and pain free. It was like I'd gone back fifteen years, before the nightmare began. My friends saw the difference in me and remarked about it often. Even today when I pass by the hospital, it does something terrible to me inside – I spent so much time there, the blackest period in my life.

My mother and the rest of the family can't believe I'm looking so well – I go walking, swimming and dancing, doing all the things I only dreamed of before.

Tony, I came to you for healing for just three months – isn't that such a short time after being sick for over fifteen years?

Today, I look at all the scars on my tummy and say, "My God! They are the reminders of that dreadful time in my life!"

It's a miracle that I'm better. Sometimes I still can't believe it!'

I have seen many people going around and around on the treadmill of life, creating the same mistakes, falling into and becoming stuck in the same self-destructive and negative patterns. They realise that something is wrong and want to make a change, but don't know how to begin. The healing they need is what I call 'self-development'.

My message is always the same. Everything in our lives is affected by how we think and feel deep within. Our inner world creates our outer reality.

So many people I have counselled have told me that every time they formed relationships with someone new they always turned out to be the same as the previous person.

The pattern continues – they feel used, abused, let down and depressed.

I always ask this simple question; 'What do you think you deserve?' To the person whose relationship has ended I always tell them to allow plenty of time before starting another, so that their feelings and thought patterns have time to change. If people could only see and change the negative thought patterns they carry with them, the world would be a happier place.

Joan worked as a school teacher but left her job because some members of the staff bullied her. She began again in another school and experienced the same thing happening. She left immediately and got a job in an all girls school, thinking it would be different. In less than a year, she was being bullied again.

At this stage she was on medication for her nerves and decided that the best solution was to make a new start and leave the country. Joan went to work in America. The first year was great, she found new friends.

Slowly, however, the bullying started again and the years of upset that had accumulated in her system saw her in hospital. Joan returned to live in Ireland and attended a lecture I was giving. She came for counselling and healing, and within six months learnt to change her inner thinking and emotional pattern. The changes were remarkable. She got another teaching post and was never bullied again.

As with Joan, self-development is partly to do with sorting and tidying up the past.

When it is necessary or relevant, I use my psychic abilities to bring a person back to a particular moment in their past, which is impacting on the present, to help them to change. Yet at the same time I don't believe in dragging up the past – it's not necessary to dig up a whole garden in order to remove a weed. In fact, many people I see who've been in therapy are more fragmented than when they began.

I try to build on the person's strengths and not their weaknesses, help them move forward in their lives. Some may need to think positively, while others need to develop confidence and self-esteem.

Charlie, a man in his fifties, wore a white shirt with the sleeves rolled up and beads of sweat rolled from his face on to my desk. He was extremely agitated, his eyes protruded and his body shook. I went to shake his hand and he exclaimed, 'For God's sake, Tony! Don't get me to relax. It's the bloody tension that's holding me together!'

Charlie had just come by taxi from the psychiatric hospital. His history of depression had spanned thirty years – mostly spent in various hospitals. He was stuck in a pattern of insecurity until he began to do some work on himself. After six months of healing and counselling, Charlie remarked, 'Now I can honestly say I like myself.'

Within one year, Charlie was a changed man. The hospitals were just a faded memory and he was off his medication. On his last visit to see me, he said, 'Tony, I love myself. I love life. It's like a whole new beginning.'

A physical problem might bring a person to healing, yet unknown to them, a crossroads has been reached in their lives – the physical problem is a symptom but only part of the 'wake-up call'. Being honest with ourselves will quickly get us back in touch with who we are and where we're going. Admitting we are lost can very often trigger a response from our guardian angels, thereby giving us a solution.

EXERCISE – HOW TO ASK FOR HELP

The following exercise will show you how to look for help in ways you might not have thought of. To prepare yourself, when life seems to be going wrong and everything appears to be conspiring against you, before falling off to sleep at night, say to yourself:

I am open and receptive to divine intervention.

Then follow through on being open. Answers can come in many different forms. Here are some you should practise being aware of:

- ❧ You may open a page in a book and there lies the solution.
- ❧ You turn on the radio and someone is speaking about a subject that rings true for you.
- ❧ You instinctively feel like taking action that leads to a solution.
- ❧ You bump into an old friend who gives you the advice that is the answer to your prayers.
- ❧ You wake up in the morning knowing what needs to be done.

Then follow through!

CHAPTER 8

THE HEALING OF ANIMALS AND PETS

'Animals are "psychic", they possess that intuitive knowledge that they are being helped by unseen hands, and they surrender themselves to it, so peacefully. They know.'

Sylvia Barbanell

ANIMALS CAN HAVE A POWERFUL EFFECT on our health and well-being. Just being around them can help lower blood pressure, boost our immune system and make us laugh. They exude so much love and affection that, should harm or illness befall them, the effect can be so distressing for the owner.

'My cat Petals is just not herself,' the lady from West Cork wrote. 'She seems very down and won't eat her food. Lately she's started to disappear for long periods of time. I'm very worried about her. Please, can you help?'

I've always used my telepathic and psychic gifts while healing people, but with animals my abilities are keener still. I tuned in to

Petals and immediately picked up her intense fear of a dog. I started absent healing and wrote to her owner telling her what I'd seen.

She promptly wrote back saying she didn't have a dog, there were no dogs in the neighbourhood and perhaps I was mistaken. Yet, each day I directed healing to Petals, I came up against this solid block of fear. I tuned in again to Petals and asked, from my mind to hers, what the problem was. Immediately I got a clear picture of Petals being chased around the house by a big black labrador. In my return letter I told the woman what I'd picked up, and asked her once again to please check it out. A week later she wrote back saying she'd recently hired a new housekeeper who had her own key and let herself in each morning, while she visited her sister in hospital. One morning she returned early to find the housekeeper's black labrador running excitedly around the house with poor Petals terrified out of her wits. The housekeeper no longer brought her dog to the house. The riddle was finally solved.

An animal can be a loyal friend and companion, a friend to talk to when we feel alone.

Peggy was attending me for healing; she had severe bronchitis and persistently suffered from migraine headaches. One evening she told me she was very upset about her dog Bobby – he was very ill and the situation seemed hopeless. Bobby was a five-month-old wire-haired terrier. He was nervous and frail when Peggy got him and wasn't getting any better. He had twelve different illnesses, the vet said, including distemper, an infectious and often fatal disease of animals. Bobby also had tonsillitis and conjunctivitis. The vet tried everything but said that Bobby would have to be put down. Peggy writes:

'At the time I'd been going to see you, and I spotted an article in your waiting room about absent healing. So I placed Bobby on your healing list on a Monday. By Friday he'd improved so

much it was like a miracle had happened. The vet had given him up as a lost cause, but the effects of healing were immediate! The infections cleared over a few weeks and he began putting on weight.

He's a strong fellow now and no longer afraid of going out. In fact he can't wait to get out the front door. He runs down the road pulling me along with him, the brat! Thank you for all your help, both for myself and my dog. That absent healing is powerful stuff!'

I'm constantly struck by the beautiful auras animals have. They appear translucent, almost angel-like. Kathleen, a blind woman, brought her guide dog, Flossy, for healing. Flossy was a beautiful yellow labrador. She'd had a serious stomach operation six months before, but the wound wouldn't heal. Her vet wanted her put down and Kathleen's heart was breaking at the thought of losing her. Flossy's aura was a sunny bright yellow, which means she was trustworthy, friendly, loyal and full of love. I knelt down on the floor as Flossy lay on her side for me and sure enough I could see an eleven-inch open wound on her stomach, oozing pus.

I placed one hand just over her wound and the other on her head and gave her healing. Flossy licked my hands in appreciation. I stood beside Kathleen and gave her healing to help disperse the shock and trauma I knew she was feeling deep inside. They went off, delighted with themselves.

'Well, Mr Hogan,' she said when they returned the following week. 'I was telling your patients outside about Flossy. The vet couldn't believe it, the wound has all dried up and is healing at long last.' I had a quick look, the infection was clear and the wound hardly visible. Flossy leaned over and gave me a big wet lick. The cloud of depression over Kathleen's head had gone and so had the shock. She found my hands and held them tightly: 'God bless your hands, Mr Hogan,' she said. 'You've given Flossy and me a new lease of life.'

A woman phoned me in a blind panic. She owned a very successful stud farm with many horses. I tuned in to one of her horses and saw in my mind's eye a vivid picture of him looking poorly, lying on the ground. 'He's been like this all week,' she'd said. 'The vet's come and gone. He doesn't hold out much hope.' I told her I'd already started healing on her horse and would continue until I heard from her again. 'He was poorly, even last year,' she explained. 'We checked his blood daily and it wasn't right, so we didn't race him. When he went down like that, we were at our wits' end and I've been ringing around all the other studs and a good friend recommended you. I'd be so grateful if you could help him in any way,' she said anxiously and hung up.

The phone rang a few hours later. 'I simply can't believe it's the same horse, Mr Hogan,' she said. 'He's down the fields running about. Everyone in the yard is amazed. Our vet is dumbfounded.'

I was delighted with the good news, yet still felt there was something in the horse's system, so I continued healing until he got the all clear from the vet. Time passed and the horse was finally fit to race again. I'd the joy of taking a flutter at the bookies and winning a few pounds on him!

'*No!*' I said to myself. 'I'm not going to bring that up.' Emily, a gifted music teacher in her thirties sat before me. She looked so much healthier in herself, a far cry from the depressed, tranquillised slip of a woman who had first come through my door. As we chatted I kept getting a distinct impression of a yellow canary in a domed wire cage draped in blue velvet. I told myself I wasn't going to mention it. But as the thought flitted through my mind, the words just came tumbling out, 'You don't know anyone with a bright yellow canary, do you?'

Emily stopped in mid-sentence. 'How do you know about Fred not being well?' she asked.

'Who's Fred?'

'He's my mother's canary – her darling! She's heartbroken over him. He won't eat. He's stopped singing. Ever since, I've been very worried about my mother's health, because when Fred isn't well, she isn't well. She just adores him.'

I explained to Emily how I heal all kinds of pets and animals.

'Perhaps we could try absent healing on Fred?'

'Would you?' she asked hopefully. 'It's been a dreadful worry. I can't wait to tell my mother.'

A few days later I got a phone call from Emily and her mother. 'Fred woke us early this morning singing his heart out! He's back to his old self. We are so relieved. Thank you so much.'

I've only to walk into a strange house and the family pet will usually make its way towards me – they sense when someone will be kind to them.

The cat will end up sitting on my lap, the dog will crouch at my feet, looking for attention. It can be embarrassing sometimes when an animal tells me to inform their owner when something is bothering them – such as wanting a different kind of food or they are being mistreated in some way. I try to be as diplomatic as I can and just make a few subtle suggestions.

Children are highly attuned to their pets and very often sense if something is wrong with them. Sam reminded me of the famous TV dog – Lassie. He had the same colouring and was so aware of everything I said and did. Sam's owner tells the story:

'My children were very upset about their dog, Sam. He was in severe pain after a car hit him on the road and he lost his appetite to eat. We took him back and forth to the vet for months but he just wasn't the same. The children were very upset to see him in agony like that. We were all upset. The whole house was upset.

One of my children, Sara, whom you treated some years ago, came to me and said, "Why not bring Sam to see Tony? He made my asthma go away." Indeed, she was right! But I'd completely forgotten about it, yet was sure that you couldn't help animals. So I kept passing it off until my husband finally asked, "Why not phone the man – for Sara's sake?" Well I felt a bit stupid but went ahead with it anyway and we brought Sam in the car to see you. As we passed your waiting room, the look on everyone's face was just hilarious. You put your hands on Sam's back and gave him healing – this was amazing because he wouldn't let anyone touch him there, not even the vet. His back healed after that one visit to you. He's now eating like a horse, or should I say like a normal dog, again. My children, especially Sara, send a special thank you.'

Animals can sometimes be a positive force for change in our lives. I was recommended to Alison's mother because Alison wasn't doing well at school.

'My mother sent me. I've a head cold and sinus,' she whispered as she sat hunched up in an anorak zipped to her chin. There were big black rings under her eyes; she looked like she could do with a good night's sleep, she let out a few yawns.

'How's school?' I asked.

'All right.'

'Have you got exams coming up?'

'Yes, my junior cert.'

It was a touchy subject from the start I knew, her mother had said on the phone, 'She's the worst in the class. Please do something with her!'

I told Alison simply what I did. Then – as I was about to put my hand on her head, she produced a large white rabbit, from inside her anorak. 'Do you heal animals?' she asked with a grin. I'd seen rabbits being pulled from hats before, but this was ridiculous!

'What's his name?'

'Roger. He's got a sore eye and a cut on his ear where the cat scratched him. It won't heal.'

'We'll see what we can do,' I said and gave them healing.

The following week Alison told me that Roger was doing fine – simultaneously producing two gerbils from under her anorak. 'Do you heal gerbils?' she asked. The more I laughed the more Alison's whole face lit up. From then on Alison brought a pet animal each time she came. One day I asked her what she'd really like to do if she did well in school. 'I'm a complete dunce,' she said. 'I only want to work in a sweet shop.' Despite what she said, I could see she had real potential with animals and told her so. Alison continued coming for healing and got the highest marks in her class, the highest marks ever recorded in her school. She went on to become a veterinary nurse.

I've been asked umpteen times to help a nervous animal when its owner is going off on holidays and leaving it with a neighbour or putting it into a kennel. Animals are so sensitive they can anticipate when their owner is going away, many weeks beforehand. Horses, too, can feel great tension and stress when confined to a horse-box for long periods of time. One woman in England frequently asks for absent healing for her horses when they're going on a long aeroplane journey to such races as the Melbourne Cup in Australia or the Kentucky Derby. She always finds they remain calm and perform well on the day.

EXERCISE – HOW TO HELP YOUR PET OR ANIMAL TO COPE WITH A JOURNEY

If you have an animal or a pet that's stressed about going to the vet or on a journey, you can really help them by practising the following exercise with them:

- Sit down quietly with the animal.
- Rub its coat slowly but firmly. Make a conscious effort in your mind to connect with the animal.

❀ Visualise a warm, loving glow coming from you to the animal.

❀ Talk to your pet in reassuring tones. Tell them simply what's going to happen. These are the kinds of things you could say:

🐾 To a cat or dog – 'I'm taking you in our car to the vet. You're going to be all right. The vet is my friend and your friend and you'll be relaxed when he gives you your injections to protect you from colds and flu through the winter months.'

🐾 To a horse – 'I'm taking you in your horse-box to the show/races. You've been there before and you're going to be fine. When we get there you'll love the whole sense of freedom and will enjoy performing. You're a great horse, a beautiful horse.'

CHAPTER 9

HEALING THE IMPOSSIBLE

'In a gentle way you can shake the world.'

Mahatma Gandhi

EVERY DAY PEOPLE ASK ME for the impossible. There have been times when I wondered how much more could I cope with, dealing with so much grief, sadness and despair, from morning to night listening to the horror stories, the heartbreak, constantly switching from one world to the next. There were times, I admit, when I found it all too much. In the early years I was constantly on the go, running from one hospital to another. I became a familiar face in all the main hospitals in Dublin. Cars and vans pulled up on the street outside my clinic, even the odd ambulance with a sick patient who couldn't make the stairs. So I healed people where they were, in their cars on the street. One afternoon, an angry woman shouted down the phone at me, 'You healers are all the same, you just don't care about people.'

'What's the problem?' I asked calmly.

'It's my best friend, she's in hospital dying of cancer of the spine. I've been in touch with several healers and they just fob me off. They won't put themselves out. I suppose you're going to tell me the same – that you're too busy?' I asked what hospital her friend was in, explained how busy I was all day and night with appointments. However, I said, no matter how late I'd finish that night, hail, rain or snow, I'd be there for her friend. Eventually she calmed down.

No sooner had I put down the phone when another call came through from a well-known publisher in America. A man introduced himself and explained that they had just published a book by a British healer and had received a call from a woman in Ireland who had read the book and whose friend was in hospital with spinal cancer, 'So we gave her your name and telephone number and hope you didn't mind' he asked.

'That's OK,' I replied. 'She has already been on to me a few moments ago by phone and I'm going into the hospital tonight after work.' We said our goodbyes and left it at that.

I finished healing at eleven o'clock that night, grabbed my coat and absent healing book and made straight for the hospital.

A thick, dense fog descended quickly as I drove, the visibility was nil. I nearly turned back but for the promise I had given the woman on the phone. Slowly I turned the corner into the long driveway that led up to the hospital, relying on memory from previous visits to guide me there. Usually there were two large white pillars on each side of the entrance, but because of the thick fog they were nowhere to be seen. I got out of the car and reached out to feel for one of the pillars. Off in the distance I heard footsteps, but the fog was too dense to see anyone.

I continued walking carefully with my hands outstretched, touched one of the pillars, then moved across the road in a straight line in an attempt to find the other one. Once I gauged where the two pillars were, I got back into my car and carefully drove through the gates into the car park. Sitting in the car I closed my eyes and asked for assistance from my spirit friends, to help me heal the woman I was about to meet.

When I opened my eyes I could just about see the soft glow of the lights coming through the windows of the hospital. I looked at my wristwatch. It was half-past eleven. I got out the car and braced myself to see if I could find the front door. With hands outstretched I stepped forward at a snail's pace. I looked back only to see that my car had completely disappeared into the dense fog. 'Right,' I said in my own mind, 'I'm here to help this woman, I promised I would come.' Through the glass door I could see the porter sitting at his desk reading his newspaper. I opened the door slowly and all the fog and mist came in with me. It was like a scene out of a Boris Karloff movie. All I was short of was the long black cape.

'You're working late,' the porter said. The place was completely empty.

'I'm sorry, I won't be a minute,' I replied as I raced up the long marble stairs to the dimly lit landing. Everything was still, there was nobody about, everyone seemed to be asleep in their beds. Straight ahead there was one door open. I walked into a room in complete darkness. I could see an empty bed on my left, a chair and a bedside locker. The woman's not there, I thought. I walked back out on to the landing. All the other doors were closed.

How am I going to find this woman? I wondered. Her friend will go berserk if I tell her I didn't make it. I tuned in to the sick woman and asked my spirit friends what to do. Immediately, I felt a strong urge to go back into the empty room. As I did, a woman's loud voice spoke, 'Who's there, who's that?' I looked up to where the voice was coming from, towards the ceiling.

'Are you the man I've been waiting all day to see. What kept you?' the angry voice demanded to know.

She was perched like a bird in a long canvas hammock, stretched from wall to wall, above the empty bed.

'I'm in this contraption of a thing because I've cancer of the spine and I can't lie in a normal bed,' she screeched, resentfully.

153

The room was in total darkness except for the dim light coming in from the landing through the open door behind me.

'Switch on the bedside light over there on the locker, til I see what you look like,' she growled as she stared down at me.

Eventually I found my bearings in the dark and switched on the small beside light.

'That's better,' she said. 'Now pull up the chair there and tell me all about yourself, are you any good?'

I didn't answer her exacting questions. I was too exhausted and shattered after a long day of healing.

I pulled up the chair and sat beside the empty bed, and every now and again I looked up and caught a glimpse of the woman's head as she edged out over the side of the hammock.

'I'm on the strongest morphine injections to kill the pain and they're not even dulling the damn thing,' she rasped. 'They said they've tried everything. It's the blasted pain. I'm in complete agony with it. I can't even go to sleep at night with the dreaded pain,' she moaned.

In my own mind I tuned in to her spirit and opened up the channels of healing to her as she continued speaking.

'Open the drawer there in my bedside locker and take out a book. It's about a woman healer in England, I've been reading it all week. It's fascinating. My friend Diana who telephoned you this morning has been trying to get in touch with the English healer for weeks, she even telephoned the publisher of the book in America.'

I found myself saying out loud, 'The woman healer couldn't come tonight so they sent me in her place.'

'Oh I see!' There was a sharp disappointment in her voice as she continued with her line of questioning. 'Do you ever get any results? Have you ever written a book? I never heard of you before, are you long doing this type of work?' She went on and on.

I could feel the anger rising up in me as she continued. I glanced down at my watch; it was heading for twelve o'clock.

When she finally stopped quizzing me I stood up on the edge of the empty bed and awkwardly ran my healing hands along the outside of the canvas hammock in line with her spine and gave her healing. I stepped off the bed to the floor and said, 'I'll be off now.'

'You won't leave me like this, will you? Will you come again to see me? Will you come tomorrow? Will you promise me?' she moaned.

At that time of the night I couldn't think straight. I told her I had appointments, all day every day, but I would try and come to see her tomorrow during my lunch-break.

I headed down the stairs and out into the cold, foggy night air, completely exhausted.

The following day, I returned to the hospital at one o'clock. It was a beautiful sunny day. I had a quick drink of water for my lunch, allowed twenty minutes to run in and out of the hospital and back to my clinic for the next appointment. I took the hospital stairs two at a time. When I reached the woman's room the door was still open. To my surprise it was full of people sitting around in a circle with notebooks in their hands, talking. I stood at the door looking in. My eye was drawn to the woman sitting in the middle of the circle, the same woman I had seen the previous night. She sat on a chair talking and laughing to all the people, with not a bother on her. My attention was suddenly broken by a voice behind me. 'Can I help you sir?'

I quickly looked around. It was one of the nurses.

'Are you looking for somebody?' she enquired.

'Yes' I said, pointing. 'I was here last night seeing that woman who is sitting in the centre of the room.'

'Oh, you're the healer we were told came last night.'

Before I had time to say anything further, the nurse continued, 'Well as you can see there's been a big turn about. She slept great last night and the pain has completely eased. Will I tell her you're here?' she asked.

'Please do.' I said and waited outside the door.

The nurse returned, 'She's having a meeting at the moment with her business managers. She told me to ask would you come back another time, she's too busy at the moment to see you.'

'I'll be back tomorrow at the same time,' I replied.

The following day I returned to the hospital at lunch-time. The same kind nurse appeared when she saw me and said, 'Oh she's just gone off to some posh place on a business lunch.' Looking at her watch she continued, 'She'll be gone for a few hours, will I tell her you called?'

Once again my heart sank having come especially to see her. The nurse sensed my upset and came closer and said, 'How can you bear to do this kind of work, when people treat you like that? All the doctors here can't believe the improvement in her. It's certainly down to you, ever since you came to see her that night,' she smiled. I thanked her for her kind words and dashed back to my clinic for my next appointment.

I was only in the door when the phone rang. It was the woman's friend, Diana, who had originally asked me to see her.

'I kept my promise,' I said. 'I've been to the hospital every day to see your friend and I believe she has improved.'

She stopped me in mid-sentence. 'Yes,' she said curtly, 'I've already heard you've been to see her but there's really no need to go and see her any more. I've finally secured an appointment for my friend to see this really good healer in England, the woman who wrote the book on healing.'

The words of the nurse rang true, 'How can you bear to do this kind of work?' The phone went silent.

The time came when I needed to stand back from my work, to take stock and see where I was going. I began to write about my experiences and to ask my spirit friends for advice. I quickly realised that there were people who were negative about my efforts to help them. The more I gave, the more they took. I decided only to work with those who appreciated what I did for them. I don't think that people fully realise the enormous sacrifices and effort that healers go through in order to heal the sick.

I remember a thin little girl from the country whose name was Maureen. She was wrapped within a ball of darkness and couldn't speak or respond. The light had gone out of her eyes a long time before. Maureen looked like somebody from a concentration camp, her spirit was broken. She was no more than thirteen years of age and had a very thin frame, just skin and bone, with dark brown hair and eyes sunk deep in her head.

I tried speaking to her to reach her but she was too far gone. All I could do was place my hands softly upon her head and ask God and my spirit friends once again for the impossible. Beneath my hands I could feel only a flicker of light coming from deep within her. The healing power flowed through me as waves of love and light pouring deep into Maureen's whole being, into her spirit. Through guidance from my spirit friends I had been told that physical healing was not possible but the healing of the spirit was, so I did my best.

Maureen's uncle and aunt, whom she was staying with in Dublin, explained that she was the eldest in the family and had brothers and sisters who lived in the country. She had done rather badly in her exams so her parents threw her out of the house, saying she was a bad example to the others in their schooling.

'We have no children of our own,' said the aunt. 'We got a call from the local police asking would we take her in. So we did. My husband and myself got her into a school here in Dublin and she's been struggling ever since. She won't eat anything. So we have to take her to the hospital every morning so that they can feed her. You are our only hope Mr Hogan,' she pleaded.

Maureen was one of my first anorexic patients. Anorexia was unheard of at that time in Ireland. Nothing much was known about the disease. Each time Maureen came, she refused to speak or respond. I continued to give her healing and eventually she began to look brighter. Her spirit, I was told by my spirit friends, had been brought back to life. Then one day, out of the blue, she whispered something as I was healing her.

'I hate the hospital, I hate the hospital, I hate going there,' she said.

'What goes on in the hospital?' I asked.

After hearing herself speak, Maureen became self-conscious and retreated into herself.

I broke the silence and said, 'I won't tell anyone I assure you.'

There was another long silence. Maureen looked up at me and whispered, 'They hold me down and put a brace on my head and chin, then they turn a big screw and force me mouth open.'

'Why do they do that?' I asked.

'To feed me,' she replied.

Tears welled up and rolled down her frail cheekbones. 'I miss my brothers and sisters,' she cried out and burst into tears.

It is at times like this, I feel put to the pin of my collar to know what to say or do. I tuned in to my spirit friends for help and just as I did I heard the words coming out of my mouth, 'You will indeed meet your brothers and sisters again, you have done nothing wrong. Your aunt and uncle love you very much.'

She brightened up and began speaking to me about her school and all her little worries and fears.

I reassured her as much as I could and was happy that we had freed her from her trauma.

Maureen continued coming to see me for another while. Her hospital visits became less frequent. She began eating again, settled into her school and made new friends. I never saw Maureen again, but often wondered what happened to her.

There are times when I feel angry at the dreadful injustices and experiences that people are going through in their lives. I got a phone call from a senior nurse who worked in the local hospital, who regularly sent people to me for healing.

'Tony, I have a woman here with breast cancer who's scheduled for radiation treatment. She's very upset and in quite a distressed state. If I put her in a taxi could you possibly see her this morning?'

Immediately I tuned in to the woman and knew she desperately needed to come.

'Of course, send her straight away,' I said.

Twenty minutes later the taxi arrived. A very frightened woman in her forties walked in. She couldn't talk, but just kept crying. I fetched her a glass of water and some tisssues. The colours over her head were blobs of dark blue and red, which told me that she was depressed, isolated and full of fear. I sat beside her with my eyes closed and asked for healing to come to her as she cried intensely from the deepest part of her being. A few minutes went by and the room began to fill with peace and light. Her crying eased and became softer. I slowly opened my eyes, to see all her colours glowing brighter and more vibrant.

'Can you talk?' I asked her quietly.

She raised her head and slowly looked at me.

'Only if you wish to, please take your time.' I assured her.

She took a sip of water from the glass.

'I won't ask your name or address or where you've come from. Please understand, I'm only here to help.' I said.

She spoke for the first time. 'I come from the west of Ireland and live on a farm. I've never been to Dublin before. I'm so afraid.' Tears welled up in her eyes again and steadily streamed down her face.

'I understand, just take your time.' I responded.

After a moment or two she steadied herself. 'I found out I had cancer a few months ago. My doctor told me I had to go up to Dublin for radiation treatment. I'm terribly afraid. I don't know anyone here.' Her voice trembled with intense fear.

'You haven't told anyone?' I asked.

'No, I've two young children, a boy and girl. I miss them so much – I'll never see them again,' she cried.

I held her hand in mine and asked my spirit friends for help for this poor woman.

'My husband is a farmer and we live on the farm with his mother. I just couldn't tell them, I couldn't tell anyone,' she cried.

'Will they not miss you at home?' I asked.

'No, I told them I was coming up to Dublin to stay for a few weeks with a school friend I haven't seen for years. I've never been to Dublin before. I'm really frightened, I miss my children so much. I'm afraid I'll never see them again.' She cried her heart out.

'It's no shame, let it all out, you'll be all right.' I said reassuring her.

All the emotions were screaming through her body, trying to find expression as her face changed from bright red to white. She gathered herself and continued.

'I'm staying in a bed and breakfast near the hospital. I'm terrified,' she screamed. 'I'm going to die. I'll never see my children again. I'm all on my own.'

'Remember that kind nurse who sent you to me, she is your friend, and I am your friend,' I reassured her. I stood up and gave her healing and soon she settled into a womb of peace. Then I sat down again.

'What did they do in the hospital this morning?' I asked as she gathered her thoughts.

'They marked the area where the cancer was, and then I was told I've to go in tomorrow morning for them to start the radiation treatment.'

I explained briefly how spiritual healing is wonderful in helping people through their radiation or chemotherapy treatment. I suggested she come to see me every day for healing, which she did. Every day the kind nurse in the hospital phoned and kept me informed as to how the she was doing. She even took her to her own house for an evening meal and took her into town on the weekends.

Under healing the symptoms of sickness and other side-effects from her treatment were considerably reduced and her frame of mind was growing stronger by the day.

The weeks flew by and finally she went home on the train to her husband and children, a different woman. I never knew her name or where she lived, but I often thought about her and wondered was she able to talk to anyone about her true feelings.

Of course, there are always the funny moments that help me to keep everything in perspective and carry on with my healing work.

Valerie came to see me one day saying, 'I'm going to divorce that husband of mine, I just can't stand him any more.'

'Why?' I asked.

'Because he's just too smelly, I just can't stand the sight of him near me.'

'Has he been like that for long?'

'It all happened about nine months ago, ever since he went to that dammed doctor.'

'What happened?'

'My husband Tom has had asthma and eczema for years. He heard about this medical doctor in one of those big posh places who told him he had allergies to water and ever since he hasn't washed himself.'

I burst out laughing.

'It's no joke Tony, even the children at home can't stand the sight nor the smell of their father. They leave the room when he walks in. Even his colleagues in work have been getting on to me about the dreadful smell and his hair looks a bloody disgrace!'

My mind went back to a man who I had treated many years before who suffered from asthma. He was told that he had an allergy to dust and to get rid of all the carpets, chairs, curtains, beds, clothes etc. Even the poor cat had to go. Eventually all the man had in his living room was a television and a wooden orange box to sit on, and a mat in the corner for his bed. Here was another similar story.

I explained to the woman that her husband couldn't have an allergy to water because the human body is made up of water.

'Can you save our marriage?' she replied.

It was then I realised how serious the situation was.

The next week Tom, her husband, came to see me for healing and the first piece of advice I gave him was to go home and wash himself. Their marriage was saved and his eczema healed.

When I first began healing I didn't have a phone. People just came on spec and queued in the hallway seated on a long line of chairs.

One morning a lot of people arrived together. I couldn't help but notice one young man with a bad limp who sat at the end of the queue looking quite dejected and depressed. In my mind I said to myself, 'I hope I can do something for him.' When it was his turn he slowly stood up with great effort and limped into my room and sat down on the stool. The colours around him were thick blobs of dark murky blue. He told me his sister Mary had recommended me to him. I wrote down on his file his name, address and all the relevant details about his health, etc. I asked about his bad leg and what happened to it.

He said he had been in a car accident the previous year and hurt his back and damaged his left leg. Everything was going just fine until I stood up and placed one hand on his head and the other on his lower back. Suddenly he jumped up to his feet like lightning and recoiled from me, shouting, 'Is this not the insurance company?'

'No,' I said. 'I'm a healer and I was just healing your back.'

He quickly moved towards the door, 'I thought you were taking down all my details to give me a quote for car insurance, my sister recommended you!'

Only then I realised he was in the wrong building; the insurance company was two doors down. Somehow I suspected that he really was in the right place, but didn't realise it.

Another time, after I got the phone put in, it rang and an anxious young woman asked, 'Do you make house calls?'

'What's the problem?' I enquired.

'It's my father, he has bone cancer. All the family came together to send him to Lourdes. But when we phoned up, we were told Lourdes closes for the winter. We are very upset and disappointed but thought the next best thing is yourself.'

In all my years of healing, I never thought I'd see the day when I'd be put in the same bracket as Lourdes!

There were funny moments and sometimes scary moments. Tom, a big red-haired giant of a man, came to see me about his wife, Angela.

'She's the problem Tony. She's just not right in the head.'

'What's wrong with her?'

'Well if you look out your front window you'll see what I mean.'

I pulled back the lace curtain and glanced out the window. The traffic was flowing, people were walking along the footpath.

Cars were parked on both sides of the street. Everything looked pretty normal to me. I turned to Tom and said, 'Where's your wife, Angela?'

'There she is.' Tom pointed his finger through the curtain.

Directly below the window, Angela was hunched on all fours like a dog. She was running around the parked cars, hiding from people as they passed.

'Tony, she's completely depressed and paranoid and on a rake of bloody tablets. I tried several times to get her up the stairs to see you, but she just won't come.'

'Have you taken her to the hospital?'

'She's been in every bloody hospital in Dublin and some of the ones up and down the country. I don't know what to do any more, I'm at the end of my tether. The past few months, she's been to three different psychiatrists and only got out of the last hospital two weeks ago.' He said desperately.

'What did they say the problem was?'

'She's depressed, obsessed, paranoid. They said she's got every bloody mental problem that's going.'

I kept glancing out the window at Angela.

'The first psychiatrist we went to, Angela thought he was the singer Alvin Stardust and attacked him. The second psychiatrist was Gary Glitter and she attacked him too. Then the third one was the Pope, so she had to be locked away in a padded cell. The worst part of it all is, when she sees someone who looks like her brother Vincent she gets very violent. She really hates that brother of hers.'

Alvin Stardust, Gary Glitter, the Pope and now her brother! I nervously asked Tom what her brother Vincent looked like.

'It doesn't matter, Tony. Depends very much on the mood she is in. She just hates her brother with a vengeance. It brings out a violent streak in her, so it does.'

Was this going to be my lucky day? I wondered.

Tom kept a constant eye out through the window while talking.

'She's moving,' he shouted. 'I better go and see if she will come up and see you.'

'Don't worry if she won't,' I called out as Tom raced down the stairs like a greyhound.

A sea of heads turned towards me in the waiting room. 'Next please,' I called out. A frail old lady slowly rose to her feet with the aid of a walking stick. She had come all the way from County Wicklow. When she was settled, I asked, 'How can I help you?'

'It's my heart, Tony, I had a heart attack about two years ago and haven't been well since,' she said and burst into a fit of coughing. I rubbed her back for her and soon she settled down again.

'At the moment I've got a bad dose of flu on me.' Just then the door burst open and there stood Tom's wife Angela. She was breathing heavily and her big, dark almond eyes glared through me like laser beams.

'Do you know that woman?' The little old lady asked hesitantly.

I kept looking at Angela.

'Is she your wife?'

A thought flashed through my mind: was I Alvin Stardust, Gary Glitter or the Pope? Worse still, was I her brother Vincent? I had visions of skin and hair flying around the room.

Angela stood at the door glaring at the two of us with a look of disapproval. Her breathing grew more intense. Slowly she stalked across the room like a bull ready to charge. I braced myself while glancing out the corner of my eye at the old woman who was look-ing back at me in shock.

Suddenly, Angela made a dart for me and shouted, 'Elvis, Elvis, I love you Elvis!'

She began running her fingers through my hair while kissing my face.

'Sing me a song, sing me a song Elvis,' she implored and as she leaped into my lap, the chair buckled and we both went to the floor with an almighty crash.

The old woman nearly had another heart attack as she jumped off her chair, ran out the door like a bullet, shouting, 'A mad woman is attacking Tony inside!'

All I could think about was thank God I wasn't Vincent the brother! Angela's husband Tom ran panting up the stairs to rescue me and took Angela away still shouting, 'Elvis, Elvis, I love you Elvis.'

I composed myself and straightened out my shirt and tie and picked up what was left of the chair. The old woman came back into the room for her walking stick, 'Tony does this happen to you very often?' There was nothing I could do but laugh.

Through my healing gifts I find it easy to spot someone who is suffering from depression, whether I am walking down a street, on a bus or in a restaurant. They all have the same qualities in their aura.

The mind energy is always dark and fuzzy, creating an overload of energies surrounding the head, which puts pressure on the brain.

A senior psychiatrist came to see me with his wife Mary. He said, 'Over the years many of my patients have been to see you with depression and I must admit I don't know the first thing about what you do, but I have seen incredible results. My wife has been suffering from dreadful depression for a very long time. I've brought her all around the world with me on lecture tours to see if any of my colleagues could help her, but so far there has been no improvement at all. She can't eat, and as you can see, she has gone to below five stone. All she does all day is to curl up into a ball and sit on the floor in a dark corner, behind the hall door. We have two lovely children and a good marriage.'

The doctor continued speaking as I tuned in to Mary. She sat completely wrapped in a blanket of darkness. There was no light in her spirit; effectively she was dead inside.

My spirit friends came around her. I placed my hands on her frail body and the response to my healing was immediate. The darkness that had engulfed her slowly began to lift and disperse. The psychiatrist stopped talking and stood back across the room with his arms folded, observing everything that was happening. The connection of the healing power had been made through my hands to her spirit.

Within the space of a few minutes everything had brightened and the whole room brightened up. Mary's stooped and twisted body responded and she raised her head and looked at me. Her face broke out in a thin smile. 'Thanks,' she muttered. Her husband spoke, 'I've seen with my very own eyes what you did. I don't know what you did, but you did it.'

The excitement built up in his voice until he couldn't contain himself any longer. He went over and kissed his wife on the lips. The evidence was there for all to see, Mary had responded to the power of healing and looked animated.

'We will come back next week Tony, if that's all right with you,' he asked happily, looking like a man who had just won a million pounds.

Mary came to see me for a few more visits and asked, 'Do you think I would be able to go to the country for a long weekend with my husband?'

'Of course.' I said, reassuring her.

The following week Mary and her husband presented me with a beautiful piece of Waterford crystal glass and a card from their two children, which read 'Thank you for giving us back a new mummy.'

The first stage in healing depression is to unblock the thick dark blobs of compressed energy that I see surrounding the head and shoulders, putting pressure on the brain. This done, all the mental and physical pressure is lifted. The electric fields start to vibrate freely again – pulsating through the whole person; 'I feel the weight of the world has been lifted off my shoulders' is a common response.

Sitting on my desk is a beautiful porcelain red-breasted robin. It came in the post with a card from Rita, a schoolteacher from County Kerry. This is her story:

'It was the 3rd of January when my life took a turn for the better. I had discovered a man who had the power to heal people. I was at the lowest point in my life. I had been consistently depressed and limp for years.

The depression, I remember, was gradual at first, then got worse. I just couldn't function at all, and the longer it went on the more it took over my whole life. Every day I was constantly living in a complete fog of negative thinking. Physically I always had a knot in my stomach and a lump in my throat. My appetite for food ceased completely. At first I thought my depression was due to a recent bereavement, but as time went on I felt myself slipping into a big black hole.

With the little energy I had, I struggled through the day consumed by negative thinking, finding myself all the time in negative situations. Somewhere, in a part of my mind, I was aware that I was losing more and more control over my life, but I didn't have the strength to prevent it and found myself becoming more isolated. I was just existing on the edge. I remember thinking to myself "If someone would come and give me a pill that would give me a quick, painless easy passage out of this black hole I was existing in I gladly would have taken it." I was on the last rung of the ladder and alas time was running out for me.

I had promised a good friend, however, that I would get on a train and see you in Dublin. I remember that morning very well. I tried to get on the train but I just couldn't, I was too down in myself. Then I heard my friend's voice in my mind saying, 'Go on, go on, it's your only hope.' I took courage in hand and stepped onto the train.

I reached your clinic by taxi and sat in the waiting room. I was surrounded by a big, thick black fog of depression. I braced myself so that I wouldn't cry. I was just one big tear drop walking around. You called me into your healing room; there was a beautiful feeling of peace and stillness in there. I sat down and I said nothing. You spoke and I listened. You told me everything about myself, all the things that happened to me in my past; what I was experiencing every day, even to my deepest thoughts and feelings. I was dumbfounded. You told me about the knot in my stomach and the lump in my throat. When you finished speaking you put your hands on my stomach and throat. At first I experienced this incredible calmness within myself and gradually all the numbness began to leave me. The knot in my stomach vanished the moment you took your hands away. The lump in my throat seemed to pulsate for a few moments, then it softened and cleared.

It is the 2nd of March now and all my depression has gone. I'm living in the day, and back to work. I love getting up early in the morning with the birds singing outside my window. Everything holds pleasure for me now; instead of just hanging on to the edge with my eyes closed I have let go. I can fly.'

EXERCISE – HOW TO GET BACK IN TOUCH WITH YOURSELF

If you're at a crossroads in your life and don't know which way to turn, try doing some of the following:

- Plant some flowers in your garden.
- Read a book that holds good memories for you as child.
- Take a leisurely walk beside the sea or through a wooded park.
- Breathe in the fresh air. A brisk walk brings you into the present moment.
- Listen to a song or a piece of music that reminds you of a time when you felt a sense of peace and freedom.

Then, write down on a page where you think you are blocked. Jot down all possible options to help you unblock yourself. You may find your way becomes clearer.

CHAPTER 10

VITAMIN & MINERAL ADVICE

'Let your food be your medicine and your medicine be your food.'
Hippocrates

HER WHOLE FACE was black and blue; one eye was so swollen you could no longer see the iris. Although Grace was in her seventies, she looked like she'd gone ten rounds with Mohammad Ali.

'Everyone keeps asking if it was my husband that did it,' she joked, her sense of humour shining through despite everything. 'It's not the first time, Tony,' she explained. 'It happened before when they changed me medication.'

The problem was her blood pressure; for over thirty years now she'd been inside most of the hospitals in Dublin. The poor woman rattled off all the medications she'd been on and was attending the hospital every week. Her recent change of medication had caused her to fall yet again and hit her head on the pavement. She was terrifed of it happening once more, being carted off in an ambulance, unconscious, into hospital.

As Grace spoke I caught the vivid image of a large jug and heard my spirit friends say, 'She's utterly dehydrated, get her to drink some water!'

'I couldn't be!' she said, her voice and hands trembling, 'I drink twenty cups of tea a day!'

'Precisely,' I replied and explained how the tablets were already having a diuretic effect on her body. Combined with all the tea she was drinking, which had a diuretic effect in itself, she was losing too much fluid. I gave her healing and got her to drink a large mug of water. As she was saying goodbye I requested in a note that she ask her hospital to check for dehydration.

On her next visit she looked so much better; she had her old confidence back, her skin was healthier, the bruising had subsided.

'Tony – you're better than any X-ray machine,' she laughed. 'Usually I never get to see a doctor. But when I asked them to check for dehydration, the doctor saw the results and asked to see me personally.'

'Missus!' he said. 'You're terribly dehydrated and before you leave here, I want you to drink at least three pints of water!'

On her next visit to the hospital Grace's blood pressure had stabilised, for the first time in many years, and her falling episodes had ceased.

I've worked as a naturopath for over thirty years now, studying the mind, emotions and how the body's chemistry is affected by what we eat and drink.

During this time, I've accumulated a vast knowledge and under-standing of vitamins and minerals, and how a deficiency can affect someone throughout their life.

For example, hyperactivity in children can be a nightmare for parents. A nervous, jumpy stomach can play havoc with a teenager's confidence. Sinusitis causes many people to feel depressed and despondent. The following are just some of the remedies I use every day in my clinic. The list is intended only as a guide. Please see your doctor or health professional first, before trying any of these remedies.

SUGGESTED REMEDIES

ARTHRITIS

There are many forms of arthritis and only general advice can be given. Drink a few glasses of water each day to improve circulation and to break down acid crystals. Take cod liver oil in the morning to build flexibility in the joints. If your joints are swollen, take a supplement of soluble vitamin C daily. Rub warm olive oil into and around the affected joints.

Avoid sugars, tomatoes, salt, oranges, marmalade and all acid foods.

BACK PROBLEMS/TENSE, TIGHT MUSCLES

Tiger Balm's intense heat stimulates the circulation and is most effective in freeing up painfully tight and tense muscles. It's made from aromatic oils: peppermint, clove, menthol, cajeput and camphor. (Cajeput is an anti-inflammatory oil from the East Indies.) There are two kinds of Tiger Balm – red and white. Red is hotter than white.

BLISTERS/STUBBED TOE

A woman who'd been visiting Australia stubbed her toe in a sliding door while out shopping. The skin peeled back and became very tight and sore. For four weeks she was unable to put on a shoe. None of the usual creams worked and the pain was immense. When she phoned I suggested she rub olive oil on the wound to help expand the skin. The relief was instant. She could wear her shoes almost immediately.

Within two days the wound was better – she was in holiday mode once more. Olive oil has wonderful healing properties. It helps with water blisters, broken skin, scraping around the finger-nails or chafed hands due to friction.

BRITTLE NAILS
Nails reflect the condition of the bones and nerves. When nails are brittle and break easily, it can signal a lack of calcium. Take a calcium supplement called cal/mag (calcium and magnesium). Rub warm olive oil into and around the bed of the nail, be it finger or toe-nail. This is a good therapeutic treatment as it helps stimulate nourishment into the nail bed.

TO BOOST YOUR IMMUNE SYSTEM
Take soluble vitamin C every day. Get plenty of rest by going to sleep early in the winter months. Spend time every day in natural light. Take ten drops of the herb echinacea once a day in a glass of warm water.

Avoid stressful situations.

CONSTIPATION/UPSET BOWEL
Constipation can be caused by insufficient fluid. Stools become hard and dry. Assuming you've already been to see your doctor, you can help yourself by drinking plenty of water daily.

While water assists the bowel to work, it can't function properly without the water-soluble B vitamins. Take vitamin B complex every day. This helps to bring fluid into the bowel.

I also recommend yogurt and a course of acidophilus to improve intestinal bacteria and break down food more effectively. Pears are wonderful because of their high fibrous and water content.

Avoid stodgy foods, sugars, chocolate, white bread, biscuits, colas and other fizzy drinks.

COLDS/BOUTS OF SNEEZING/SORE THROAT/RUNNY NOSE
At the first sign of a cold, take zinc lozenges. These can be sucked

in the mouth and are effective in shortening the life of a cold. Zinc also helps to speed up the healing process after an operation – the effects of burns etc.

Signs of zinc deficiency are: loss of fertility, poor mental awareness, low resistance to infections, poor healing.

COLD SORES
Take a course of the amino acid lysine. Rub a small amount of yogurt every few hours into the cold sore.

DRY SKIN
Drink plenty of water during the day if your skin is dry or flaky. Apply Bach Flower Rescue Remedy cream to the affected area.

DRY/DULL/LIFELESS HAIR
Your hair reflects your overall health; if you're losing your hair, you must improve your diet. Eat nourishing foods rich in protein and iron.

- *To strengthen/thicken hair:* break an egg and rub directly into your scalp. Leave it there for as long as possible, then shampoo as normal. You'll find your hair is much thicker as a result.
- *Dry/flaky scalp:* use pure coconut oil. Melt the jar of coconut near a radiator or over steam, then rub it into the scalp. Again, leave it for as long as possible. Shampoo as normal.

ECZEMA
Eczema very often disguises a nervous disposition caused by a lack of calcium. The most obvious sign of deficiency is when you hold your hands out in front of you, and they begin to shake. I recommend a daily calcium supplement to build up the nervous system. Evening primrose oil is also very effective in treating dry and itchy eczema.

Avoid salt, bananas, oranges and sugar.

EYE TWITCH

This condition is often called a jumpy nerve and can be very irritating. The remedy is a daily supplement of B vitamins.

Avoid foods that destroy your nerve vitamins, such as alcohol, cola and sugar.

EXAM STRESS

Many parents have found that calcium is excellent for children who are sitting exams and it helps poor concentration, irritability, sleeplessness, nervousness, bad temper and panic attacks. Calcium takes a few days to penetrate the system – it depends on the levels of depletion. You might also try Bach's Rescue Remedy, which helps to calm the mind and body. Take four drops in a small amount of water four times a day.

Avoid stimulants, alcohol, coffee, sugar and chocolate, and all fizzy drinks that contain caffeine.

INSOMNIA (MILD)

Take a drink of camomile tea with a spoonful of honey. This helps to calm and soothe the nervous system. Another excellent herbal remedy for more chronic insomnia is avena sativa. Add a few drops of this herb into a warm drink before retiring.

Avoid tea or coffee late at night, sugar, chocolate and cheese.

LEG CRAMPS

Take a calcium/magnesium supplement. Massage your legs with olive oil to improve circulation. Try and go for a walk during the day.

MENOPAUSE/HOT FLUSHES

Common symptoms are sudden sensations of heat in the face and upper body. Sweating and patchy redness of the skin follows, together with night sweats and interruption of sleep. I recommend a glass or two of soya milk daily. Vitamin E and a calcium/magnesium supplement are also helpful.

Avoid salt and all foods containing salt.

PREMENSTRUAL TENSION/SYNDROME

Take a course of evening primrose oil, vitamin B6 and calcium. Eat calcium-rich foods such as parsnips, turnip, honey and porridge.

Avoid sugars and sweet foods, spicy foods, wine and chocolate.

SORE THROAT

Gargle with warm water. Add lemon juice to cut through the phlegm. Repeat this a few times a day. Before going to sleep at night, mix a spoonful of honey with a slice of lemon in warm water. Sip it slowly so that it softens the lining of the throat.

SLUGGISHNESS/LISTLESSNESS

If you feel tired or sluggish upon wakening, drink a glass of warm water when you rise and another before breakfast. Add a slice of lemon, which will help cleanse and break down toxins that have accumulated in your system overnight. Try it for a week and notice how your energy levels improve.

STIFF JOINTS

If you suffer with stiffness in your knees or elbows, or they make cracking noises when you bend or stoop, rub warm olive oil on the area before going to bed. Overnight, the joints will soak up the oil and this will help to improve circulation. Take some cod liver oil.

STOMACH BUG

Take natural yogurt with acidophilus. Drink a few glasses of flat lemonade. Take sips of water throughout the day. When you start to feel better, eat bland foods such as chicken and rice. Take a supplement of vitamin B complex.

Avoid tap water, milk, cheese and eggs.

SUNBURN
Dab some cider vinegar on to the affected part. Or, better still, have a cider vinegar bath. Gently rub aloe vera into the skin.

Eat a meal that's full of protein. This helps the body heal the affected area.

If there is shock, take Bach's Rescue Remedy, four drops in water four times a day.

THRUSH
Take a spoonful of yogurt, which contains live cultures, every few hours. In addition, take a supplement of acidophilus, and cut out sugars and alcohol for a while.

TIRED FEET/BUNIONS/CORNS/ATHLETE'S FOOT
Soak your feet in a basin of warm or cold water – depending on your preference. Add a half-cupful of cider vinegar. Soak for twenty minutes. Place your feet on a towel and allow them to dry naturally. This treatment stimulates and energises your whole internal system. Finish by rubbing some warm olive oil into your feet.

URINARY TRACT INFECTION
Though more women endure this infection, men can suffer with it too. Repeated courses of antibiotics don't seem to be a lasting cure for this ailment. I've found the following treatment is most effective. Empty a cup of pearl barley into a pan of water and boil slowly. Allow to cool, then drink the juice; adding a drop of lemon will help make the urine acid.

For a more potent effect and to improve the taste add some cranberry juice to your barley water.

EXERCISE: HOW TO COMPILE A DIET HISTORY

If you want to find out what foods you might be allergic to, try the following exercise. Write out your diet history for six days. What you'll need is:

* An A4 sheet of paper. Divide the page into three columns, headed Breakfast, Lunch and Tea, working from the left.
* Twenty minutes after each meal, jot down all the foods you've eaten, including sweets, snacks, drinks, cigarettes, chewing gum, etc. Make sure you note everything down. Do this for six days.
* Then go through your list with a pen. Pin-point the foods you've eaten most commonly over the six days. Select one food item and try to stay off that particular food for a week to see if your allergy symptoms go away.

People who try this exercise have been astonished at the amount of sugar, salt, soft drinks, alcohol, chocolate and spicy foods they've eaten in those six days. They hadn't realised, for instance, that they drank so much tea and coffee every day. This exercise often led to a change in their eating habits; the result was a healthier body and a happier mind.

CHAPTER 11

DOES HEALING ALWAYS WORK?

'Something we were withholding made us weak until we found it was ourselves.'

Robert Frost

IT'S HIGHLY UNUSUAL to come for healing, even for a short period of time, and not receive some benefit. The improvements can be seen: in a better quality of sleep, increased energy levels, pain is eased, a troubled mind set free. These significant changes show that healing is having a positive effect on the patient's whole being. Of course, if a person has had many operations, it can influence the effectiveness of healing.

A middle-aged woman in a wheelchair had had one hundred and four operations on her back. There was so much scar tissue that the most I could do for her was reduce the pain and lift the depression that came with it. After the healing she acknowledged that the quality of her life had improved dramatically.

A young girl, one of the first in the country to have joint replacement, suffered with chronic arthritis. Operation followed operation, but the replacements weren't successful. Unfortunately

I couldn't do much for her but reduce her pain, because there was little of her left.

Not everyone is ready for healing. A husband who's browbeaten by his wife is one such example. Leo was diagnosed with bronchial asthma. His nocturnal coughing kept his wife awake until the small hours. In exasperation she told Leo she had made an appointment for him to see me – and that he was to turn up on time! Leo had no intention of co-operating. To each of my questions he replied, 'You should ask the wife, she'll tell you.' I discovered he smoked forty cigarettes a day and had no interest in ever giving them up.

His name was Peter and he wanted to know 'what I did'. Peter had been a passenger in a friend's car when it was hit from the side. The windscreen smashed and they both landed up in hospital.

'How's the driver?' I enquired.

'He has a bigger claim in than me!'

'Is he seriously ill?'

'No, no – just a bad back like mine. He's the one that told me about you, but he won't come himself in case you fix his back too quickly!'

'Oh, I see!' I replied.

'I wouldn't mind coming in about six months – after my insurance claim is fixed up in October.'

There was no point in talking. I stood up to give him healing.

'No! I don't want you to do any of that healing on me,' he insisted.

'I'll just place my hands on your head, to take away the shock I see in your system,' I reassured him.

'No – I don't want that either. It might affect the results on my neck and back!'

'I won't touch your neck or back,' I promised.

He eventually agreed. The healing flowed through my hands. I could feel it calming him within. Suddenly my concentration slipped when I felt him move his hands suddenly to his face.

'What's that on my face?' he gasped. I leaned forward and saw blood trickling from his forehead.

'Don't rub your face!' I cautioned and quickly fetched tissues and a mirror. The healing had effectively pushed out the glass that was embedded in his head. His knuckles were also bleeding, where the glass had popped out from beneath the skin. We counted out forty-nine shards of glass on to a sheet of newspaper.

'They told me that they'd removed all the glass in the hospital,' he complained.

'And that the tiny scars would heal in time! It's no bloody wonder my face has been paining me for so long!'

I tried to explain, almost apologetically, about the healing, but Peter was so shocked by its immediate effect, that he blurted out, 'I definitely won't be coming to see you now. Not until the insurance money is secured!' He moved towards the door and quickly vanished.

There are also those who I describe as 'doing the rounds'. These are the hypochondriacs – as soon as I heal one complaint, another set of symptoms arrives. Before seeing me they'll have seen someone else. After seeing me, they'll be off again – doing the rounds.

Some people can actually seem ungrateful for the healing they've received. Tom was a lecturer in a Dublin college, highly motivated and ambitious. He drove himself hard and frowned on those who paced themselves.

A keen rugby player when young, he expressed his competitiveness on the playing pitch, later honing his ambition at work. He was highly paid and travelled the world on lecture tours, jetting from country to country like some human whirlwind. Then one day the whirlwind stopped, and Tom's world came crashing down around him.

He discovered he had myalgic encephalomyelitis, chronic fatigue syndrome, more commonly known as ME.

Tom had just turned forty when he first came to see me, and had all the classic symptoms of ME; his physical strength was nonexistent, completely drained of energy with pains and weakness in every muscle, depressed, forgetful, disoriented, chronic flu-like symptoms and constant sore throats. Tom had schoolmates who were doctors, who prescribed medications in an effort to keep him going. But his whole system rapidly shut down.

He couldn't work or drive his car and was stuck in bed for two long years. When I'm healing someone with ME, it can take a superhuman effort to kick-start their immune system and get them moving again. Tom was no exception. His energy level was zero. I would flood him with healing energy and watch it come and go like a weak glimmer of light. Tom was of no help to me at all. He lived in his head and was full of intellectual theories. I tried and tried again, eventually making a connection. At last his body kicked into life and off he went.

The following week, Tom returned chuffed with himself. He'd driven home to see his mother, a hundred country miles away, he said. He was back at work, had given two lectures that week and stayed up late writing class notes. His concentration and memory recall had returned.

I knew by his attitude that he was going to use up every drop of energy I'd given him. I continued with his healing, however, until his ME symptoms diminished. He continued pacing himself like a top athlete – cramming in lecture tours to France, Spain and Germany, returning to me shattered, depressed and complaining. I cautioned him about conserving his energy, but it was like talking to a brick wall.

Eventually, Tom became too busy to come for healing and fitted me in when he felt like it. I hadn't seen him in a few months when one morning he stumbled in the door, coughing and sneezing, his clothes and hair covered in dust.

'I'm no better!' he wheezed. 'I've been coming to see you for the last few months and look at me! I'm wrecked! I've no energy. I've pains all over – your healing isn't working!' he ranted.

'What have you been doing with yourself?' I asked. 'You look a right mess!'

'I bought this bloody three-storey house, and I've discovered the roof's riddled with dry rot!' he moaned.

'It'll take a fortune to fix – but to save money, I went ahead and took the roof off myself. The carpenters are coming this afternoon,' he said with relish.

I went silent – checked the address on his form and tried to contain my anger.

'Tom,' I said, 'you live in a three-storey mansion, and you're telling me you removed the roof: joists, beams, slates – the whole lot by yourself?'

'Yes!' he said proudly. 'It took a solid week, working all day and through the night, but I got it done in the end. It'll save me a fortune!'

'But it'd take twenty men to do what you've just done!' I said. 'And you're telling me my healing didn't work!'

I couldn't believe what I was hearing and showed him the door.

As I have said, some people are in denial, out of touch with their true feelings and not ready to be healed.

'Are you under any stress?' I asked Ann-Marie simply. Ann-Marie was a nurse who suffered with dreadful back pain and migraine headaches.

'No!' she said, as she moved off her chair and sat on another.

'Do you suffer from tension?'

'No – I'm very relaxed. All my friends say how relaxed I am.' Ann-Marie moved to another chair.

'Are you worried about anything?'

'No – my mind is worry-free,' she said and yet again moved to another chair. For a brief moment I thought she was playing musical chairs! Then she turned to me and said 'Good God, is that the time? I left my washing on the line,' and took off out the door like a bullet.

When a person is out of touch, it can take a great deal of patience, time and counselling to help them recognise they have a 'problem'. For example, healing won't magically transport someone from a bad marriage, which can be the underlying cause of an illness. When someone expects instant miracles I ask them to wait, while I get my magic wand from the bottom drawer! If nothing else it gets a good laugh.

A person can become ill because it gives them a measure of control and, once they've discovered this control, the last thing they want is to give it up.

Mrs Sheen's daughter wheeled her mother into my healing room, then waited with her two sisters outside. Mrs Sheen was in her sixties and crippled with arthritis. I could see from her aura that I was up against it, but I gave her the opportunity to come around.

'How can I help you?' I asked.

'Help me!' she snapped. 'If only I was young again! My husband Oliver is dead many years, and I've had to bring up my three lovely daughters all on my own,' she moaned, her voice full of resentment and bitterness.

'I live all alone in a big house; they have a great life and look at me! I used to go dancing, swimming and travelling the world,' she said, looking down at her trapped body in the wheelchair. 'Why did this happen to me?'

I quickly realised it wasn't her arthritis that needed healing, but her extreme negative attitude.

'How can I help?' I asked yet again.

'What are you going to do for me?' she growled.

Why bother answering someone who's so self-centred and negative, I thought to myself, and placed my hands on her knees. As I moved quickly to her feet, a feeling inside told me there was something wrong. I asked my spirit friends for advice and clarity. *'She's faking it!'* came their blunt reply. I immediately took my hands away.

'What's wrong?' she asked irritably. I stood back and had a long look at her aura.

'What's wrong?' she repeated.

Looking directly into her eyes, I said, 'Exactly – that's just it. There's nothing wrong.'

'What do you mean?' she barked aggressively. 'How dare you! I'm crippled with arthritis, just ask my doctor.'

'You may have arthritis, Mrs Sheen – but there's strength in those legs and you can walk all right,' I said.

She was taken by surprise, so stunned, that she fell silent for a few moments. Then her voice softened and she said meekly, 'You've found me out ...'

'But why are you doing this?' I asked.

'It's my way of keeping the family together. You won't tell them, will you?' she implored. Nimbly she got out of her wheelchair and beckoned me away from the door, in case her daughters outside might hear what she was saying.

In hushed tones she told me how, in the daytime, she would abandon her wheelchair and walk around the house. With her daughters at work, she'd slip out – always taking different routes to the library or a shop where nobody knew her.

If the need arose she'd keep her daughters on their toes, telephoning them at home or at work, rushing them back in the evenings to attend to her every beck and call. She wouldn't allow them a holiday, to go anywhere without her, not even a day out. Her so-called arthritis was a tool to control their lives.

I told her that she was a very selfish woman, that her daughters' happiness was just as important as her own needs, but she refused to listen.

'You won't tell them I'm a cheat?' was her only concern. I could see that all three daughters adored her, that I was in a 'no-win' situation.

Like an actress changing roles, she jumped back into her wheelchair and headed for the door. Outside, stood her three faithful daughters.

'Are you all right, mother?' one asked.

'He can't do anything for me,' she growled. 'I'm too far gone. I knew I shouldn't have come here. Let's go home.' Her daughters looked at me with some puzzlement, then wheeled her away.

Healing can be a second chance, an opportunity to make changes, to put right the wrong, to get one's life together. I'm very conscious when this special moment happens – the power and strength of healing is felt immediately. I've met many who've lived terrible lives, but through some traumatic experience were given a second chance. I call this a spiritual awakening.

It was late one cold winter's night as I stepped from the bus into sheets of torrential rain. I'd been called to the bedside of a woman on the outskirts of Dublin.

'You're drowned!' the daughter said and ushered me into the hall.

'Come into the kitchen, I'll get you a towel to dry yourself.' When I'd finished, she brought me to the living room.

'Mammy's in here,' she whispered and led me into a darkened room where an elderly white-haired woman lay in bed.

'I'm sorry for bringing you all the way out here,' the woman said. 'It's such a dreadful night.' I shook her hand and immediately felt she hadn't much strength left in her body.

'Call me Hannah,' she said feebly. 'The family had to make a bed for me here. I can't climb the stairs no more.'

I pulled up a chair as Hannah told me her life story. She was a kind, sensitive soul who had had a very hard life and confided in me about the burden she carried. An air of sadness filled the room, as the rain pelted the window pane.

'Would you go over to the mantelpiece and get me my rings?' she asked. As I brought them to her, she tried fitting them on to her fingers, but they, and her wrists, were badly disfigured and swollen.

'They've been like this, ever since I got the cancer,' she said – her voice lowering to a whisper. 'If I could only die, Tony, with the rings on my fingers. Do you think you could help me?' she pleaded.

I told her I would do my very best for her.

As I started healing, a beautiful feeling swept into the room. The presence of Hannah's mother and late husband were standing beside her.

I reached over and put my hands on Hannah's stomach and head and gave her healing. As she lay in bed with her eyes closed, her appearance took on a new life – she looked radiant. I sat back in the chair and let my spirit friends continue their work. Twenty minutes passed. Hannah awoke with a smile on her face. 'It's beautiful, Tony. My mother and my husband Tom are here.' she said.

'Yes, they're here Hannah. I see them,' I answered, as tears of joy trickled down her face.

'When you first put your hands on me, I felt myself coming out of my body. I went into a place where all these beautiful angels were. It was magnificent. Members of my family, who'd died a long time ago, appeared and told me they'd been helping me all along. I was to let go of all that was upsetting me down the years. I was told I'd been given a second chance.'

The healing that night had a profound effect on Hannah. She was relieved of her burden.

The following week she herself opened the door to me. She showed me her hands. All her rings were on her fingers, the swelling had gone and so too had her bed downstairs. A totally changed woman, she was full of plans for the future.

EXERCISE – HOW TO ACKNOWLEDGE YOUR HEALING

If you are in the process of getting better, the most important contribution you can make is to acknowledge your healing on a daily basis. Those who fail to do so can quickly slide back into negative cycles of despondency and despair – focusing more on getting worse than getting better.

Acknowledge the good inside yourself. This expands your positive mental attitude and brings good feelings to the fore, which create the right chemistry in the body and mind towards getting well.

- In this exercise, daily, write in your diary the improvements you've felt, no matter how small they are.
- Express the improvements to yourself and to others.
- Have patience with yourself. Look forward to the time when you are completely well.
- Write your healing story in letter form, and give it to your healer or therapist. They, too, need to be acknowledged. This is the encouragement they need to help you and to continue to help others.

CHAPTER 12

ABSENT HEALING

'The efficiency of Absent Healing is proved when there can be no other possible explanation for a sick person, whether recovering from a physical or mental disorder, making a recovery – partial or complete – from the time the healing intercessions have commenced on that patient's behalf.'

Harry Edwards

I DIDN'T KNOW HOW IT WORKED or why it worked, but it did. It all started when I first began healing on my travels around the country. A scribbled note slipped into my hand spoke of silent suffering; people trapped behind their four walls at home or others fighting for their lives in hospital, or a child awaiting a major operation.

A friend or relative would slip a hastily written note into my pocket before I left town. Scribbled writings on cigarette packets, backs of envelopes, pieces of cardboard or paper napkins, would all tumble out of my pockets on to the bed. Exhausted though I was I would muster up some strength from somewhere and concentrate on those sick people to ease their burden, lift their fear or remove their pain. An image would form in my mind as I tried to imagine a light flowing from me to them across many miles to a darkened room or a hospital ward.

Days would pass, sometimes weeks or months, but eventually someone would tell me that the patient had improved or made a remarkable recovery. Sometimes relief was given. 'All the fear left her Tony,' an old man once cried as he shook my hand. ' She passed away peacefully.'

Now, every morning as I begin my healing work, letters arrive from all over Europe, America, Africa, Canada and Australia. From the four corners of Ireland they come; people whom I've never met, never seen nor heard of before.

They write requesting healing for themselves, a family member, a friend, a neighbour or a workmate. Many are in constant pain with shingles, a slipped disc, angina, emphysema or cancer.

They seek relief from alcoholism, vertigo, depression or bereavement. 'My best friend has lupus,' one wrote. 'A teenager is in a coma.' 'A child has behavioural problems.' 'A young mother has a brain tumour.' 'There's been a death in the family.' Or this:

'My friend Joanna is only twenty-six years of age. She has three young children. Two weeks ago she was diagnosed with breast cancer. She is so upset, worried and full of anger; completely devastated by the news. Over the next few weeks she will have her right breast removed, Tony, and some of her lymph glands. The thought of her disfigurement has severely depressed her. After the operation, she faces months of radiotherapy and chemotherapy. Joanna really doesn't deserve this – she had just got her life back together, after her marriage failed. Please, Tony – could you help her?'

The tone of each letter tells its own story. With some, the writing is hard to make out, yet I feel sufficiently in tune to know they badly need my help. Some in old age are frightened of dying.

Unbeknown to them, a friend will seek healing on their behalf. Absent healing is often requested for a person who is mentally disturbed. Nurses have sought healing for a patient in their care; for someone in a bad car crash or a sick child who cannot speak for itself. Here's an example:

'I had a call one afternoon to say that my nephew's little boy – Adam – of eighteen months had been dragged out of a pond in the garden, black and not breathing. They were in Liverpool. He had been rushed from one hospital to another and put on a life-support machine. They brought his breathing back. But there wasn't an awful lot of hope. We were panic stricken. Adam was packed in this ice apparatus with monitors and six needles dripping various drugs into different parts of his body. On the third or fourth day, the doctors came to his father and said, "Would you tell everyone to stop praying. There are worse things than death." He would be a cabbage; he would be blind and he probably wouldn't be able to speak at all. So we were quite devastated. The little child – no life ahead of him. My first thought was to put him on absent healing. I contacted you – because you were the last hope we had really. The day after he was put on the absent healing, he suddenly started to move his arms.

That was the first movement, the first sign, and then later on in the evening he started licking his lips. I think it was the next day or that night, he suddenly opened his eyes wide and indicated he was hungry. It was just unbelievable! The doctors came in, they just couldn't believe it, the nurses all gathered around the little boy.

Adam didn't know what had happened to him at all. He couldn't remember anything. But he was able to talk at least, he was able to see. And the next day, one of the nurses took him out of the bed – the parents still stayed with him – and he ran up and down the ward. People just couldn't believe it. When the doctor who'd been caring for him walked in, he said, "I cannot believe that this is the same child. It's just a miracle!" And that's what I believe it was. We all believed it was just a miracle. The child is now thirteen years of age. He's doing extremely well at school and has a great personality and sense of humour. It's just ended so well for us.'

Late in the evening, when everything is quiet, I open my healing request book. It contains a list of those who have requested healing – either for themselves – or for a friend or loved one. Beside each name is a photograph with an outline of the person's general condition and illness. I close my eyes and attune myself to my spirit friends and to God, the source of all healing. An impression immediately forms within my mind of the person I wish to heal; intuitively I have made contact. I feel their presence and what they are experiencing. I begin to project healing energy to them, as well as asking my spirit friends to administer corrective healing for their particular ailment or need.

Healing begins from that moment on. The link has been established, and it will continue on throughout the day and during the hours of sleep – boosting a depleted system, calming a troubled mind, easing pain, reducing anxiety and fear.

Absent healing is a great friend in times of stress, anxiety or worry. It can help with the stress of sitting an exam, the fear of flying or going to the dentist, or the trauma felt by a young child just starting school. It has helped those laid low with a debilitating illness, such as a severe dose of flu. It has eased the stress of those moving house, getting married or retiring from work.

'After my dad retired he got so bad with stress and tension that he seemed unable to cope with day-to-day affairs. He fussed and worried over the simplest of things, and his negative state of mind caused him to have many sleepless nights. He simply could

not adjust to his retirement. As his only daughter, I felt so broken-hearted seeing my dad – whom I loved so much – become so helpless. Having been to you myself for healing, with marvellous results, I put my dad on your healing list.

Almost overnight, he began to improve. Initially, he became very calm and relaxed.

He was back in control of his life. His old sense of humour returned. He even took a long weekend away in the country, which was totally unheard of previously.

It's as if he became child-like again; carefree in his attitude towards everything.

It's difficult for me to find words to describe the complete change in him. But the whole family are delighted to see him back to his former self again. My dad doesn't even know he has been helped by your healing gift. If I told him – perhaps he wouldn't even understand.

But he would certainly agree it worked for him.'

Absent healing is different from hands-on healing. There is no physical contact made. The 'healing projection' lasts a few seconds, minutes or even longer. Its progress and effectiveness can be traced back to when the healing request was first received and acted upon.

'I am pleased to relate that, since last Wednesday, my mother has a much improved state of mind. Her depression has almost gone. Her physical condition has improved greatly. As you know Mammy's condition is due to a very serious operation. Part of her stomach was removed, with her spleen and part of her bowel. As a result she eats very little and suffers with dreadful nausea, but since last Wednesday this has improved!

Prior to our neighbour placing Mammy on your absent healing list, she was very depressed and weak, unable to pick herself up. Thankfully, due to your healing efforts, Mammy has come along great. Please continue to help her and I'll let you know how she is progressing over the coming weeks.'

Absent healing has helped many when facing stressful and anxious situations. Actors have requested healing for their big opening night; the anxiety of a job interview; the stressed out woman expecting her first baby; the attack of nerves before giving a speech or a presentation; anxiety pending a court case or a driving test.

From all the letters I've received down through the years many have found absent healing to be marvellous in helping them through their chemotherapy and radiotherapy treatment. A noticeable feature is a speedier recovery time and fewer side-effects.

Absent healing is requested primarily in letter form. The letter tells me about the patient's illness and story; how it began and how it has advanced.

Whenever possible, I ask for a photograph of the person who needs my help. This allows me to tune in to the patient more easily. When I receive the letter and photograph, no time is wasted – healing is sought immediately for the sick person.

Within a couple of days of absent healing commencing I will reply personally to confirm that absent healing has started, with a leaflet outlining how it works. In my letter, I will explain how important it is to keep me informed of any changes as they occur. The person who places another on absent healing acts as a vital link between the patient and myself. They are my eyes and ears, as it were. They help me maintain a purposeful healing to the patient. A small piece of information, however irrelevant, can be vital to the person's recovery.

A woman in her eighties wrote to me from the west of Ireland, W.B. Yeats's county, County Sligo. She had been laid low in her bed with a chronic chest and sinus infection. She had been on numerous antibiotics for well over a year.

When she first wrote, I could hardly make out her letter; her writing was just a mere scribble across the page. On her second letter the improvement was reflected not only in the dramatic change in her handwriting, but in the whole tone of her letter:

'Thank you Tony for your letter confirming that I am on your absent healing list. Well, you will be pleased to learn my chest infection cleared up a few days after you said you started. At long last I can breathe in air again!

The sinus infection is gradually improving with each passing day. I'm certainly beginning to believe in absent healing. I must try and get rid of this negative attitude and have a more cheerful outlook on life. Thanking you most sincerely for your efforts in helping me.

I'm looking forward to paying you a visit soon to thank you personally.'

In order to keep my absent healing files organised and structured, patients are placed on my healing list from one month to the next.

I file away those who have made a full recovery, and concentrate on those patients who are in need of constant healing.

Healing energies will continue to the sick person every day, for a whole month. If a person wishes, they can renew the request for another month, and continue for as long as it takes to overcome the problem or illness.

Numerous people can be placed on absent healing at any one time. A family member may request healing for their whole family going through a crisis or for some neighbours. A woman from near Zurich in Switzerland writes with a progress report on more than twenty people from her village.

When people from another country travel to see me for contact healing, they frequently request absent healing as a follow on. For example, Rosemary had travelled from Scotland to see if I could help her. She had been suffering with chronic flu-like symptoms for over a year. Antibiotics and steroids followed one another with little or no effect. She had to go into hospital for a series of tests.

Finally, a psychiatrist diagnosed her condition as reactive depression, and put her on anti-depressants.

'If only I could get a lift. Feel a little better,' she kept repeating while telling me her story. Rosemary looked pale, listless and worn out. She spoke in a whisper, as I sat right up close to hear what she had to say. She hadn't slept in many months and her loss of appetite was evident as her bones protruded from her face.

I gave her hands-on healing, and suggested she place herself on my healing list. Later she wrote to me.

'Tony, I promised to let you know how I've been feeling since I visited you two weeks ago. Well, I'm feeling so much better now! Life has become very pleasant for me again. My sleep pattern has improved considerably. I'm now getting a very restful night's sleep and I'm waking up refreshed. The awful depression lifted a few days after my visit to see you, and I'm able to concentrate once again. I am happy to say I'm back reading the newspapers, watching television, paying attention to my appearance. Thank God, and thank you.

I must say I'm having the best week's health that I've had all year, and feeling much more positive and optimistic now, facing into the winter. I'm actually feeling "physical tiredness" now, something that had eluded me for ages. Please continue sending healing to me through your healing prayers; there is no doubt that I can feel your healing presence helping me every day. Many thanks for all your help and kindness.'

Whenever I get a few moments of quietness during the day I seek healing for those who are in need of immediate help. This I call my 'emergency absent healing list'.

It may be a crisis phone call – for someone undergoing a serious operation, in a car accident, a woman who is expecting her baby within the hour, a person close to death.

'I am writing to let you know how your absent healing treatment worked on my fourteen-year-old godchild. Last Sunday week, Matthew developed what appeared to be the beginnings of a cold. He collapsed in school the next day and was brought home.

The following day, Matthew was brought to the doctor who diagnosed pneumonia and recommended a course of strong antibiotics. Wednesday evening his breathing became unstable and the doctor was sent for again. He immediately called an ambulance. Matthew was admitted to the general hospital where a battery of tests were carried out. He was diagnosed as having a rare form of viral pneumonia. Immediately he was put on stronger antibiotics, sedatives and a respirator. By Thursday Matthew got so bad he was given the Last Rites.

His poor mother and father were completely shocked at how quickly he had deteriorated. They were told that there was very little hope for him. I received a phone call from the parents telling me the bad news. Initially I went into shock. Then, I thought to myself – how can I help? Over the years I had, on many occasions, received great benefit from your wonderful healing gift. So I rang and asked you to place Matthew on your absent healing list. On Sunday morning, I rang Matthew's parents.

They said that Matthew had a very good night on Saturday. His heartbeat and breathing had stabilised, his temperature had come back down to normal. The virus that had been moving around Matthew's body, had eventually been isolated. Needless to say, Matthew's parents were extremely relieved. Today is Wednesday, and I have since learned that Matthew is much better. He was taken off the respirator. Now, he is sitting up and taking liquids and talking to his Mam and Dad.

Thank you for all your great efforts in sending healing to Matthew. I believe your healing intervention played a major part in his recovery. He was so ill on Thursday and so much better by Monday. I was so upset and worried when I heard the news about Matthew. But thanks to your wonderful work of absent healing I felt I was able to do something positive to help.'

When a family member falls ill, it can be an extremely traumatic time for everyone. The family, friends and relatives don't know where to turn or what to do.

The impact is felt like a vast ripple on water; the shock and trauma reaches all the relatives and friends of the family. I am very conscious when healing, that the positive effects of the healing also ripple out to those who are connected to the person who is ill.

Lorraine had gone into hospital for a routine check-up, when they discovered she had a massive tumour in her womb. No time was wasted; the very next morning she would have the tumour and her womb removed.

I received a frantic phone call from Lorraine in the hospital, asking me to immediately place her on my healing list.

'As I talked to you on the phone, I felt an immediate calmness come over me, an inner confidence that I had never felt before. I just knew that everything would be all right. That night I slept soundly and had a most beautiful experience: you and a number of other people stood around my bed with their hands out in front of them. A beautiful soft golden light poured out from the tips of their fingers into my body where it was sick.

It was the most beautiful experience I've ever had. The operation was a complete success. The doctors couldn't get over my ability to heal so quickly. Most of the other patients were a bit put out – that I was up and about so soon while they were still recovering.'

Lorraine went to see her GP for a check-up. He told her that, after such a major operation, a large percentage of women get depressed and end up on hormone replacement therapy. But Lorraine didn't need anything. Her GP put her remarkable speedy recovery down to her positive mental attitude. Lorraine, however, put it down to absent healing.

It's only natural to fall apart at the news that you have to have an operation. Attitudes of scepticism to healing can quickly change in such moments of crisis. One such case was John. He wouldn't come for hands-on healing because he didn't believe it would work for him. At the same time he was terrified of an impending operation. His wife, Emily, wrote to ask me to place her husband John on healing. This is Emily's story:

'My husband John, who is forty-three, has suffered with constant earaches and weeping ears ever since he was a child. Last October, our doctor sent him to an ENT specialist, who examined John's ears and said they were rotten and badly infected.

The specialists went on to say that John would need an operation and he would organise it in due course.

Immediately I wrote and asked for absent healing. Six weeks later, a letter confirmed that a bed in the hospital was available. Naturally, we were both very anxious about the whole thing. John was admitted to hospital on Thursday, to have the operation Friday morning.

I found him, early Friday afternoon, sitting in the corridor all dressed up, with his suitcase by his side, ready to come home. I asked him what on earth had happened. He said that three doctors had examined him before the operation and found his ears to be completely clear. It was a miracle!

John is normally sceptical about such things, but he certainly believes in healing now. He's even telling all his mates at work! I just can't express in words how relieved we

*both are. Thank you from the bottom of my heart for all you
have done.'*

Absent healing has also helped many a pregnant woman through a
difficult birth and the recovery afterwards.

The following was written on a 'thank-you' card from Julie, a
young woman in her twenties, who came to see me near the final
stages of her pregnancy – suffering with panic attacks and fear.

> *Just a note of appreciation for all your help and healing
> during and after my pregnancy. I found, very strongly, your
> healing powers helping me through the birth of Brian. I experi-
> enced such a peace of mind, happiness, and an inner strength
> and found the whole birth a wonderful experience; not a fright-
> ening one, as it was with my first child. Brian is doing fine now
> and thriving, I am so thrilled with him.*
>
> *I would like you to know how grateful I am to you, and
> when the weather gets a bit better, I'll call to show you the little
> man himself.'*

Babies and children respond extraordinarily well to absent healing.
Dermot, who lived in England, knew nothing about absent healing. When he received the bad news about his baby daughter he
was too upset to take anything in. So, his friend, Cathal, asked for
a photograph of her and, returning to Dublin, placed Dermot's
baby daughter on absent healing. This is his story:

> *'It was in the summer of 1982 that our daughter was born in
> Westminster hospital in London. We named her Inor. She was
> born two months premature, and as a result she had to stay an
> extra few weeks in hospital. It was then that we learned the sad
> news that Inor was born with two holes in her heart and would
> require surgery. Needless to say our whole world turned upside*

down at the very thought. She was released into our care but we would need to bring her back when she was a little older for heart surgery.

A year later we received an appointment with the special heart hospital in Kensington in London. Tests were carried out and the two holes were still apparent. An appointment was made for the operation.

One day my wife had been chatting to a good friend of ours about Inor and he said he knew a man called Tony Hogan – the spiritual healer in Ireland. Cathal asked us for a photograph and said he would send it on to you to place Inor on your absent healing list. We didn't know anything about spiritual healing or even believe in it. In fact it didn't register much in our minds at the time as we were so distressed. A few weeks passed and we returned to Kensington hospital for our appointment for the operation. The doctors carried out many tests and X-rays, but found much to their amazement that the two holes in Inor's heart were closed over. They were bewildered at this and we were completely overjoyed at the wonderful news. The operation was cancelled. Inor didn't have to undergo heart surgery and we were so relieved.

I can certainly say that the instance of absent healing coincided with the time she was found to be healed of her heart condition.'

I am sometimes amazed at the trouble people go to when requesting healing. Some will draw in coloured pencil the cartilage in their knee, which I'm to work on, or the area of their back that's giving trouble. However, there is often a funny side to the letters I receive.

Marie, from Surrey in England, asked for healing for her daughter Rosanna, who lived on a Greek island. With her next letter she included a rather large, detailed map of Greece – just to make sure I knew exactly which island she meant.

A woman from America placed her husband on absent healing for his stomach ulcer. Bill worked for an international bank and travelled around the world on business. Included in her letter was a six-months' itinerary, outlining the various countries he would visit from week to week. Of course this was quite unnecessary.

Absent healing reaches the person on the spirit level, transcending time and space. Some people wonder about the precise time I carry out my absent healing work. It usually coincides with the moment they feel the healing energies reaching them.

Pauline, a schoolteacher in her forties, came to see me on a regular basis. She had a range of physical problems and I was also counselling her over a marriage break-up, because of her husband's alcoholism.

One day, she handed me a large rolled-up sheet of paper held together with an elastic band.

She looked on smiling as I released the band, and discovered a pencil drawing inside.

'Who does it look like?' asked Pauline.

'Well, it looks like me!' I exclaimed, as Pauline laughed.

'It seems to be a drawing of me!'

Pauline laughed again and told me the following story.

Her sister, Heather, whom she placed on absent healing, was in hospital in the country, awaiting an operation for a serious bowel condition.

One night, as Heather was going off to sleep, she became aware of a man standing beside her bed, gently smiling down at her. The man placed one hand on her tummy and another on her head. Heather experienced tremendous heat coming from his hands, which was both soothing and comforting. The man then turned and walked away.

The next morning, Heather asked the ward sister about the stranger who had entered her room during the night.

She was astounded to learn that no one had come into the ward

– and no doctor was on call. Heather spoke to some of the other patients, who suggested it must have been just a dream.

As the day progressed, however, Heather felt so much better in herself and was even more convinced than ever that her experience was real. She could vividly recall the man's face. Heather was an artist by profession, so she decided to draw a likeness of him.

Pauline arrived at the hospital and found Heather sitting up in the hospital bed looking so much better. With an air of excitement Heather beckoned Pauline to her bedside, reached under her pillow and took out the drawing. As Heather began telling the story, Pauline looked down at the drawing and exclaimed – 'That's Tony!'

Heather's condition improved so much, she didn't need an operation. When discharged from hospital, she paid me a visit and confirmed her experience that night.

Many people write and describe similar phenomena. There are others who describe seeing my team of spirit healers who work with me around their bed at night.

Ken came to see me many years ago, and was healed of psoriasis – an 'incurable' skin disease. Like most people, Ken forgot about the healing once he got better. That was until he became the victim of a severe car crash, which left him hospitalised for months. Operation followed operation, but nothing relieved the dreadful pain in his back. The pain, now affecting his legs, left him terribly angry and drained of energy.

Ken was confined to bed when he came home from hospital.

As there was no prospect of him returning to work, his employers let him go. A year passed, and Ken had slipped into a zombie-like state of pain and despair, doped up with strong medication.

One day, Ken's wife Maureen, brought home a magazine and left it lying around the house.

It lay there for over a week, until Ken accidentally opened a page, which had a photograph of me inside, with an article about my healing work. 'That's the man who cured me years ago!' said Ken excitedly to his wife. He told her about his psoriasis, how it was cured before they got married. Maureen wrote immediately and asked me for absent healing to help ease Ken's dreadful pain. Two nights after I began sending healing to Ken, this was what happened:

'Because of the constant pain I was drifting in and out of a light sleep. Suddenly the room began to brighten. I lifted my head off the pillow and became conscious of a number of people standing around my bed. They all looked like doctors, dressed in white. For a moment I thought I must be back in the hospital.

But I soon realised that I was indeed at home in bed. My mind went completely still. Waves of peace spread through me, enveloping every part of me. One of the people dressed in white put his hands gently on my neck and shoulder-blades.

Another placed his hands right into my back where the pain was, and began to manipulate it. It felt like a red-hot poker, going into my spine. The heat became more and more intense, until it overtook the pain. I just lay there, looking on. It was a pleasant experience. When they had finished, one of them smiled down at me, as if to say 'There you are! You'll be fine now', before disappearing into a cloud of blue mist.

The pain in my back gradually subsided. My spine cooled. Soon there was no pain at all. I leaped out of the bed, wakening my wife in the process, and began pacing the floor. My wife thought I'd gone nuts. I kept testing my back, bending down and tipping my toes – something I hadn't been able to do for well over a year.'

Once absent healing begins, for some their progress becomes evident instantly, while with others progress can be seen over a longer period of time. Either way I like to hear back if there has been a change. Sadly, there are those who request healing, but never write back. I am left in the dark. They assume that, because

I've reached the person with the healing, I should also know if an improvement has taken place.

One Sunday morning, I received a message on my answering machine to ring a Mr Wyatt urgently. I telephoned the number that day. Mr Wyatt explained that his mother-in-law was dying of cancer; she had only days to live. She was sent home from hospital to die. Could I help her in any way? He knew nothing about spiritual healing, or how it worked, he said. But he had heard good things about me from one of my patients.

In the background I could hear a woman crying. 'My wife is here with me,' he said, lowering his voice. 'She's very attached to her mother and naturally upset about the whole situation. If it would help any to speak to her, then I will put her on?'

The line went silent. I could sense that his wife was just too upset to talk. I could hear her sobbing her eyes out.

So I explained briefly to Mr Wyatt how absent healing worked; how I never limit the power of healing, even at this late stage. The healing would help his mother-in-law pass over peacefully into the next stage of her life.

Just as I had finished Mrs Wyatt came on the phone. She told me that the doctor had given her mother only a few days to live and to make the most of it. She didn't want her mother to die any faster than was necessary, she said, as she broke down crying.

Mr Wyatt took the phone once more and asked me if I would place both his wife and his mother-in-law on absent healing to help them both through this terrible ordeal. I promised faithfully that I would, and asked him to send me, as a matter of urgency, a photograph with all the relevant details. I emphasised the importance of letting me know, either way, how things were progressing.

Weeks, then months passed. I kept my promise and continued to send healing to both of them. I received no letter or word as to what had happened. Two years passed.

Mrs Byrne, the woman who recommended me to the Wyatts,

came to see me one day. Her little nephew was suffering with a bed-wetting problem. We chatted away, and during the course of the conversation I remembered the telephone conversation I had with Mr Wyatt and his wife.

I assumed that the poor woman had passed away peacefully. So I asked. Mrs Byrne looked at me puzzled.

'Are we talking about the same person, Tony?'

'The woman who was sent home to die, I got a call …!' I explained.

'Did they not tell you?'

'Tell me what?'

'Mrs Wyatt's mother made a remarkable recovery. She's over in Spain, on her holidays at the moment. I can't believe they didn't contact you,' she said with a look of surprise on her face.

As the shock wore off, I heard myself say, 'That's life.'

As a healer, one of the most rewarding aspects of my work is the help I can give when someone is approaching death. Absent healing is a wonderful comfort to those who are passing on. It helps reduce anxiety and fear, and can limit the trauma the person may be experiencing.

Late one evening, just as I was finishing up after a hard day's work, the phone rang. At first I thought there was nobody on the other end of the line. Then I heard a faint breath, as a voice broke through the silence. It was the voice of a man, crying out in the wilderness.

'Can you help me? he whispered, his breathing heavy and laboured.

'Can you help me?' There was a long pause. Immediately, I tuned in to the man and knew he was in trouble.

'There's no need to strain yourself,' I said. 'I understand. I know you need help and I want you to listen to me carefully. I'm going to direct healing to you over the phone, and I want you to just close your eyes and try to relax for a few moments.'

I closed my eyes, and saw in my mind's eye a grey-haired man in his fifties, with big broad shoulders and dark brown eyes. I could see he had a very serious problem with his throat. A dark blanket of intense fear hung around him. I urged my spirit friends to help him, but they were already there. The healing power reached him quickly; I could feel it flowing towards him. Moments passed. I opened my eyes when I felt the healing power cease, picked up the phone and slowly asked, 'How was that?'

There was a long pause. Then his rasping voice broke the silence.

'I'm here in the hospice,' he said, 'dying of throat cancer. I've not long to live. I'm terrified of dying.'

The power in his voice faded to a whisper, until I could hear him no more.

'Don't stress yourself,' I urged. 'I understand where you're coming from.'

I went on to tell him what was going to happen during his passing – there was nothing to fear.

I explained about going towards the light, and reassured him that my spirit friends and I would be there with him, helping him every step of the way.

He began crying. Then the phone went dead. That night, and every night, I sent him healing until I knew he had passed on.

When I get a phone call like this, I pull out all the stops. Every word is important. It's as if the healing energies are wrapped around the words I speak. The right words seem to form in my mind, impressed upon me by my spirit friends.

Some weeks passed. One morning the doorbell rang. A woman had come to tell me that it was her husband, Tom, who had phoned me that evening.

'He passed away peacefully, a few days later,' she said, 'and he asked me to promise him faithfully I would come and give you this message. He wrote it all down here on a piece of paper, word for word, to tell you how much you helped him that night,' she said.

She handed me the precious little note, which read:

'I felt a great peace I never felt before, after talking with you on the phone. All my dreadful fear about death just left me. God bless you, and thank you!'

Wouldn't it be wonderful, I thought later, if I could find a more effective way of linking people to absent healing. I asked my spirit friends for help. Through them I received two powerful exercises. 'Enter the silence' and 'A healing prayer of light'. I give them to you now.

EXERCISES – MEDITATION

When you are ready, read down through both exercises until they become familiar to you. Then close your eyes and let your mind become still. Tune in to the healing vibrations that surround me and my spirit friends.

ENTER THE SILENCE
Enter the silence
Speak softly my name
Tell me your troubles
Tell me of your pain.

Speak to me of your feelings
That dwell deep in your heart
Know that I hear you
We are not far apart.

Then just be silent
For a moment or two,
So I can send healing
Directly, to you.

A HEALING PRAYER OF LIGHT

Pause for a few moments. Then, as you say the following words, visualise a brilliant white light pouring into your whole being. See and feel yourself enveloped in pure white light.

Healing light above me
Healing light below me
Healing light on the left of me
Healing light on the right of me.

Healing light behind me
Healing light in front of me
Healing light surround me
Brilliant light around me.

Healing light protect me
Healing light heal me
Healing light free me
Healing light be me.

You can practise both meditations twice daily, until they become part of your everyday routine.

CHAPTER 13

THE SPIRIT WORLD

'Do not stand at my grave and weep
I am not there, I do not sleep.
I am a thousand winds that blow;
I am a diamond's glint on snow.
I am the sunlight on ripened grain;
I am the gentle autumn's rain.
When you awaken in the morning's hush,
I am the swift uplifting rush of quiet birds in circled flight.
I am the soft star that shines at night.
Do not stand at my grave and cry
I am not there. I did not die.'

Susan E Fry

PEOPLE HAVE A GENERAL KNOWLEDGE of the basic things in life, but when it comes to the subject of death, they've been abandoned by their peers and left in a state of bewilderment and fear. Part of my healing quest has been to empower those with awareness of life and death and the spirit world; to set them free from this nightmare of confusion, trepidation and fear.

I'd been called to the top floor of Jervis Street Hospital to see a man who'd been diagnosed with lung cancer.

He lay on his bed in his dressing gown, comfortably puffing smoke from a long cigar. The narrow room consisted of six occupied beds crammed tightly together up against the wall. Tall Victorian windows looked down on to the street below. As I sat sandwiched between two beds, the man talked incessantly about his 'concerns' – the major one being his MG sports car parked below on the street.

My attention was drawn to another man who lay in bed on the other side of me. He was thin and frail and looked lost and all alone. I made contact with him telepathically and he kept his eyes glued to mine.

Beyond his bed I could see clearly the outline of a woman in spirit standing close by. She was tall and vibrant with honey-blonde hair; I sensed it was his wife. The frail man turned his head on the pillow to catch what I was looking at.

The woman looked at him with a kindly smile, then a powerful beam of white light fused with the man's aura, sending it rippling towards me and over the head of the man with the cigar whom I'd come to see. The woman beckoned him gently with her hands.

His spirit eased slowly from his frail physical body and hovered above. A nurse approached and, lifting the man's arm, began talking to him. Then all hell broke loose: the nurse shouted for help – doctors and nurses came running, pushing a machine on wheels. I was moved brusquely to one side as they applied pads to his chest and shouted 'Stand back!' They kept trying to resuscitate him. The man and woman hovered above them, looking on. A few moments later the man and woman, realising I could see them in spirit form, looked over at me. The woman smiled while the man looked a bit lost. I spoke telepathically to him and reassured him that everything was fine.

The woman took his hand and they left through a vortex of blue and white mist.

It then dawned on me that I had come to see this man to help him pass over, and not the other man with the cigar. At times like this we're always helped by close friends from the spirit world.

Just one more!' my spirit friends said. I looked at my appointments book to check whether I'd seen everyone. Sure enough I'd finished healing, so I began answering letters and tidying away files.

'*There's a man outside*,' my spirit friends insisted.

I opened the door to the waiting room and saw a middle-aged man sitting there with his eyes closed. He was immaculately dressed, in a dark navy suit and tie.

'Are you all right?' I asked.

He suddenly opened his eyes and said, 'Hello – yes I've just been sitting here for a while. I can't explain it; there's a beautiful feeling in this room. I feel better already.'

As he sat in my healing room, his sister appeared in spirit beside him. '*Tell him it's me. His baby sister, Chris*,' she said. In a daze the man introduced himself as George. 'There's one question I'd like to ask,' he said. 'It's been haunting me for months.'

'What's that?'

'Every night just before dawn I awake to find a figure sitting on the edge of my bed. When I reach out to embrace her, she disappears. It's so real – I've had the experience for the last six months. What is it?'

For a moment I didn't know what he was talking about. Then Chris came through and spoke. '*George, it's me Chris – your baby sister. Pandora is with me. She's fine.*'

I relayed the exact message to him. Immediately he broke down and cried. 'Pandora is my daughter. My pride and joy. She was killed in a horsing accident. I've never got over it,' he wept.

George mourned the loss of his daughter for several minutes, then wiping away tears asked, 'Who's the figure that wakes me up at night?'

Chris came through again. '*George – it was me trying to help you. Please don't try and do anything foolish. I love you very much.*' As I told him what I was hearing, George admitted he couldn't live without Pandora any more and wanted to end it all.

'Chris was always looking after me, all through my life. She's been my guardian angel,' he said with tears streaming down his face.

'She's still an angel,' I insisted. 'She's been helping you ever since and today she's made a supreme effort to tell you she loves you very much.'

I asked George to close his eyes and tune in to Pandora and Chris, both of whom were standing beside him.

I gave him a special kind of healing to increase his psychic sensitivity; a few minutes later a smile broke out on his face as he felt their presence. Isolation and fear had been replaced by love, and a firm and lasting connection was made. George opened his eyes. He looked animated – full of life.

'Now I know they're here with me. I can feel them both and their love for me,' he said looking ten years younger.

'I don't know how I came to you. This morning when I woke, I was in a terrible frame of mind. I went out walking, without knowing where I was going and ended up here with you. It's truly remarkable the gift you have.'

A tragic experience can shape us to see life in a different way. When a tragedy happens, I try to impart what I know about the spirit world, how life goes on and never ends.

She'd come straight from the children's hospital, brought to me by her kind neighbour. Helen was screaming at the top of her voice, 'My baby, my baby!' She then collapsed howling into the chair.

My spirit friends interceded – healing flowed. I could see a tall thin woman standing beside Helen, holding a baby in her arms. I waited till Helen drained herself of emotion. Her neighbour told me what had happened; toing and froing to the hospital with her baby, phone calls in the middle of the night. Until eventually the baby died in hospital a few hours before.

'I should have taken her home,' Helen screamed hysterically.

'It's all right. You did what was best,' I assured her. 'Tell me everything.'

As Helen told me her story, I watched the spirit outline of the woman holding the baby.

'Your baby is with a tall thin lady,' I said. 'She used to wear lavender tweed suits and loved red roses.'

'It's my Aunt May!' Helen exclaimed. 'She looked after me in Cork, when I was young. She loved red roses!'

'Your baby has passed into the spirit world and is safe with your Aunt May. May's looking after her.' I continued.

Slowly Helen's sadness and hearth-ache began to subside. I gave her healing, she felt calmer and more peaceful. My job was complete.

Five years later, Helen – who was now living in England – wrote saying she'd recently been to see a medium. She wanted to deepen her understanding of what life was all about, and had re-established the connection with her daughter and her Aunt May.

NEAR-DEATH EXPERIENCES

During our time here, we experience various aspects of life in order to develop. We come from the spirit world and return there when our time is ready. We are spirit in a physical form; the spirit world is all around us, just as TV and radio waves are everywhere. Although we are unable to see these waves, if we have a receiver we can make them visible; so, too, with the spirit world.

Many adults and children have told me of their near-death experiences – often known as NDEs. Each experience was induced by a near critical or fatal event: a car crash, an operation, giving birth, falling from a height, a heart attack, an overdose, an accident or sudden shock. Some had the experience while they were asleep or meditating. Here are some conclusions from what these people have said:

- ❧ Almost all said they didn't fear death any more.
- ❧ Most said it was a beautiful experience. They remember the feeling of rushing through a long tunnel, seeing a bright light and feeling a loving presence.
- ❧ They saw relatives and friends from the past. Others described how they floated out of their bodies – watching themselves and everything that was going on around them.
- ❧ Some saw their lives flash in front of them and were given a choice to either stay or go back to continue their life on earth.
- ❧ Many described seeing colours they'd never seen before, hearing music that was out of this world.
- ❧ For many the experience had such a profound effect it turned their whole life around. They changed jobs and began helping others; it changed their personality, they came out of themselves and were more loving to people around them.
- ❧ Connections to time or material things no longer mattered.
- ❧ The psychic, telepathic and spiritual side to their lives became more active. Many described seeing the future before it happened.

Darren was a young boy who came to me for healing. He had a rare form of cancer and experienced many near-death experiences, both in hospital and at home. His mother told me that Darren kept alluding to his Nana, his grandmother, who was in the spirit world and whom Darren said would look after him when the time was right.

He described her in great detail even though she'd died before he was born. Many times, as Darren was on the verge of death, he'd recall people his mother used to know. One was a country girl she'd lost contact with. They'd worked in a factory together as teenagers.

Darren knew her name and his mother's pet name and incidences in the factory only his mother and her long lost friend could possibly know about.

When Darren finally passed away, his mother returned to the country village in search of her friend. She was told that she had died years before – still talking about her, right up to the time of death, still using her pet name.

LIFTING THE VEIL

I've been asked many questions on the whole subject of spiritual matters and the spiritual world over the years; here are the most common ones with my answers.

Q: What happens when I die?
A: When it comes to the time of passing, we leave our physical form and return to the spirit world. Our spirit is attached to the physical by what is known as 'the silver cord'. It's an energy umbilical cord that is severed at the right moment by those who assist in our transition. These are called deliverers or spiritual midwives. We gradually lose consciousness to this world and awaken to the other world. No one is left on their own, and we meet with familiar faces, such as family members and friends.

Q: What do people do all the time?
A: Well, they don't sit around and play harps all day. They continue to develop themselves and to express their talents and abilities. Those who are evolved and have specialised knowledge assist those who are channels on earth – such as healers, artists, musicians, writers and surgeons.

Q: What does the spirit world look like?
A: It mirrors the earth. Just as there are many countries in our

world – many we may never see in this lifetime – so, too, there are many dimensions in the spirit world.

Q: What does a spirit look like?
A: It looks the same as a physical person, but in the form of a light body.

Q: What is a ghost?
A: A ghost is a spirit who is earthbound. When in physical form they weren't enlightened and as a result developed a strong attachment to material things. We often hear of them possessing an old house or a castle.

Q: Where is the spirit world?
A: The spirit world is all around us. It vibrates at a higher frequency than this world. Most people's senses are trained to see just the physical form. Yet there are those who can look beyond the physical to see the spirit aura, and the spirit world.

Q: How do people communicate in the spirit world?
A: People use their visual mind to project and receive. It's very much like the silent language used between a mother and her child.

Q: Do animals have a spirit?
A: Yes, they have a spirit and return to their own spirit world.

Q: What happens when someone dies in an accident?
A: There's a difference between enforced death and natural death. A natural death is when the adjustment is made gradually and in different stages. An enforced death is when someone passes over quickly in an accident – such as a car or plane crash. People who've been involved in accidents often recall seeing the event as if in slow motion. This can cause temporary confusion and a period of adjustment is needed before the full realisation is felt.

Q: People who've almost died – what do they mean when they say they saw their lives flash before them?

A: Every experience, thought and deed is held in the ether that surrounds us. This ether is called the aura. It's like a photographic plate and contains our life's record – our 'book of life'. As we pass into the spirit world there's a speeding up of vibrations, which changes our perception and makes our life's experience visible. Here on earth, if someone is psychic they too can read the spirit aura or 'book of life' and see the development of the soul.

Q: Why does my mother keep telling me she sees invisible people in her bedroom?

A: As people grow older they move closer to the spirit world. It can be a confusing time for them and their loved ones, especially when the older person sees spirits all around. They slip in and out of this spirit dimension, regularly saying they can see people in the house or hospital. It's sad when the only reaction is to cart them off to a mental home, when all that's required is a little understanding.

Other cultures place great importance on their elders, on their dreams and visions of the spirit world. Native Americans, for instance, accept this transition as a normal and natural occurrence.

EXERCISE – HOW TO COMMUNICATE
WITH LOST LOVED ONES

When someone we love passes on to the greater world – the spirit world – it's sad when we stop communicating with them. For their concern for us is as great as ours is for them. They're in our world as much as we're in theirs, and they never stop loving or trying to help us. Being open to them helps very much in assisting the flow of communication between the two worlds. Practise the following exercise to help you achieve this:

❧ Speak their name softly; this will help you establish a bond or link with them.

❧ Act naturally. Contact is frequently made when you're doing things as simple as hoovering or cooking a meal, or when you're absorbed in a book.

❧ Be aware of their presence. Very often it's a soft, gentle awareness of them just being there.

❧ Acknowledge the help you're receiving from loved ones who've passed on; and remember they're always trying to help us.

CHAPTER 14

THE GIFTS THAT WE HAVE

'When a great moment knocks on the door of your life, it is often no louder than the beating of your heart, and it is very easy to miss it.'

Boris Pasternak

'HAVE YOU EVER DONE ANY SINGING, or played the piano?' I asked once again. She stopped crying for a moment.

'What?' she asked in a bewildered voice. I felt foolish standing there asking these questions, but my spirit friends were urging me to probe further.

'Don't mind me crying, I'm like this all the time,' she whispered. 'I've been depressed and crying all through my life. It's like there's something missing. It's been this way all the time, ever since I was born. Nothing gives me pleasure any more,' she sobbed. Miriam was a gently spoken woman in her early forties. She'd come to me with depression on the advice of a friend. Her aura had a band of sky-blue around the throat.

'What's the question?' she asked.

I was going to let it go, when I heard my spirit friends say, *'Ask her again!'*

'Are you interested in music?' I enquired. She paused for a few moments,

'No, no – not really,' she muttered. 'I played a little bit when I was young.'

'What instrument did you play?' I persisted.

'Piano – I played piano,' she said in a broken voice. At last I knew I was on the right track.

'Why did you ask such a strange question?' she wanted to know.

'When you first came into the room, I could see you had a gift with your voice,' I offered.

Miriam was startled. 'You have a strong blue band of energy over your throat,' I said. 'I usually see this colour around people who have a gift with their voice. Have you ever thought about singing?'

'No, not really,' she said. 'I used to sing as a child, but apart from that no, not at all.'

'Well, I feel that singing is your gift,' I said as I gave her healing. 'I'm just passing on the message.'

On her next visit she looked completely different. She was full of bounce, smiling, bright and happy.

'Tony, I felt so much better after seeing you,' she said. 'I kept thinking over what you said about me having a singing voice. You know, during the week, I've been practising at home – just to hear my own voice. It was a wonderful, liberating feeling.' As she talked about singing, her aura lit up like a Christmas tree. She had come upon her gift.

Miriam continued her healing. She got a spot in a local hotel at weekends, singing a couple of songs there, but she was thrilled with this. Her healing concluded and I didn't see her for a long time.

Out of the blue, she came to tell me that she'd been singing not only around the country but in other parts of the world. Now, however, she needed healing for her nerves, as she was about to appear on television. Her television debut was a great success and two years later I read a newspaper article praising her extraordinary musical voice.

These days, far too much emphasis is placed on education and exams. I've met broken people who've 'punched time' in dead-end jobs, eventually losing all purpose and going off the rails. Many had degrees, with letters before and after their names – bank managers, solicitors, judges, doctors, teachers and dentists. The pressure of education had forced them on to a path that was against their real nature. I call this a sickness of the soul. All had been pushed into a career at an early age, until the strain caught up with them. Priests and nuns came to see me suffering with nervous breakdowns, 'My parents left me in the seminary when I was fourteen. They just wanted me in a religious order, to guarantee them a place in heaven,' is a common comment.

I believe it's important to enjoy what you are doing. Happy are the parents who keep education in perspective, who are open to other creative avenues for their children. Some show natural talent at a early age, while in others it lies dormant, only to be discovered later. I remember listening to a music teacher on the radio one evening. He said that there are parents who bring their children to music lessons and force them to practise for hours on end until technically they can play fairly well, but there's always the child who seems bored and won't practise, yet when they play the place falls silent. The music pours out of them. This is a child with the gift.

As a rule I never tell children where their gifts lie – it may impose on them an unnecessary pressure. They first need to develop their personality, friends, sport, interests, skills, schooling etc. There are however, exceptions to the rule.

A child may come to me at the right moment, just as they're going down the wrong path. It's then I point them in the right direction.

'Sit there in the waiting room,' she told her daughter. 'I just want a quick word with this man.' One look at her aura told me that this woman was autocratic, used to getting her own way.

'Alice suffers with terrible headaches,' she said. 'She's coming up to her exams and I want her to do well.'

I knew exactly what she meant when she said 'to do well'! She sent Alice in. Alice's aura was soft green, which told me she was a sensitive soul. 'You get on well with your dad,' I said. She lit up. I knew that she and her dad were on the same wavelength.

'What's happening in school?' I asked.

'I'm doing exams in the next few weeks.'

'What would you like to do?'

'Well, all the girls are either doing medicine or law. I don't know if I'll have enough marks to do either.'

'What does your mother think?'

'She wants me to be a doctor, but I don't know if I'm good enough,' she replied nervously.

I was looking at a born artist, not a doctor, but I kept quiet for the moment, healed her headaches and off she went.

On the next visit, Alice's mother appeared through the door to give me 'an update'.

'On my side of the family, my brother is a doctor, you know? I also had an uncle a doctor …' she continued, making her point perfectly clear.

Alice bounced in the door looking so much better, full of energy and confidence.

I decided to wait until Alice was fully better, before I told her what I saw – I knew her mother would be angry with me for spoiling her plans – the visits would quickly come to an abrupt end. On Alice's fourth visit, I told her what I had seen all along – she was born to be an artist. Alice lit up immediately.

As I predicted, the phone rang a few days later. It was Alice's mother. She cancelled the appointment and I was told off in no uncertain manner. The words of my spirit friends rang through, *This is part of the life of the healer.*

A year later, as I was walking along a busy street in the heart of town, I noticed a group of girls on a footpath, talking. As I passed, a voice shouted out, 'Mr Hogan!' I turned and Alice ran towards me – all smiles, her portfolio in hand. 'It was exactly as you predicted Mr Hogan, I'm in art college. I love it!' she said, beaming from ear to ear. I asked how her mother was. 'Slowly coming around Mr Hogan, but my dad is so delighted for me.'

We said our goodbyes and I walked away happy in the knowledge that my spiritual gifts had set a child free to follow her natural path in life.

Fear very often prevents us from pursuing our path of expressing our natural ability. We fear that our gift won't earn us a living, that we'll end up poor. This often goes back to our parents who say – Get a real job! There is no money in that! Take that silly notion out of your head! You'll be laughed at! You've no qualifications! What will people think?

Some well-known companies have sent me staff who were about to retire so that I could help them adjust, and find something they were once good at. I remember one man came on the recommendation of his boss. He had a year to go to retirement. I took him back over his life, as a young boy in Cork, to find out what he'd put aside in order as he put it 'to get on'. He discovered his gift was wood-turning.

Six months before he retired, he set up shop in his garage and began turning out beautiful wood sculptures and pieces of furniture. Every time he came to see me, the sheer thrill showed in his face. His physical symptoms – arthritis, asthma, psoriasis, varicose veins – disappeared overnight. His wife said she never saw him so happy and contented. It was like living with a new husband.

Your natural gift needn't be something extraordinary; it can be the simple knack of describing characters and events, later put into writing. Organisational ability, the gift of putting across simple information, can make people's lives a lot easier. The ability to reach children on their own level has resulted in people opening up playgroups. An eye for colour in art and fashion is another wonderful gift.

A woman came to see me after her husband passed away. She was quite down in herself, but throughout our conversations, she spoke of her lifelong interest in colour.

'I can see the exact colour in my mind's eye that brings out the best in a room,' she said passionately. 'All my friends ring me for advice.'

I suggested she develop her talent. She now runs a successful business in interior design and features regularly in the top magazines.

You may have spent half your life working at something that was expected of you, so in order to make a life change you must be patient with yourself, to discover the treasure deep within.

EXERCISE – HOW TO DISCOVER YOUR NATURAL GIFTS

Try the following exercise to help you discover your natural gifts:

- Ask yourself what you are passionate about.
- What kinds of books do you read the most?
- Off the top of your head write down a list of things you are good at.
- Look back over your life. What were your interests when you were younger?
- Ask a family member if they noticed in the past what talents and abilities you expressed naturally.
- Before going off to sleep at night ask your subconscious mind to reveal to you what your gifts and talents are.

CHAPTER 15

YOU CAN HEAL YOURSELF

Come to the edge.
No, we will fall.
Come to the edge.
No, we will fall.
They came to the edge.
He pushed them, and they flew.

Guillaume Apollinaire

IF YOU WOULD LIKE to help yourself heal, improve your confidence, overcome worry, communicate with your guardian angel or simply reduce stress, then try some of the following techniques that I teach to my patients.

When we fall ill we can make our condition far worse by thinking stressful, worrying and fearful thoughts. This in turn creates more stress. A whole chain reaction is set in motion, which puts further pressure on the mind and body leaving us powerless to fight back. It is well to know some of the classical symptoms of stress:

🌿 Poor appetite. Feeling tired all the time. Unable to have a good night's sleep.

❧ Suffering from indigestion. Mouth dry. Biting your nails and fidgeting. Sweaty hands and feet.

❧ You've pain in your back and neck. Feeling weepy. Dizzy and disorientated. Constantly trying to take in breath.

❧ Poor concentration and memory recall. Constipation or diarrhoea. Symptoms of a cold coming on.

❧ Headaches – described by some people as a steel band vice grip across the head.

❧ Staring into space – can't get moving. Not feeling yourself, but helpless to do anything about it.

If any of the above symptoms sound like you, then you need to practise the following relaxation technique so that it becomes part of your everyday life.

Relaxation is one of the vital cornerstones in any self-healing programme. It helps reduce stress, anxiety and negative emotions within the mind and body, thereby giving your own self-healing powers a chance to heal.

Each time you practise relaxation, you are helping your mind to shift away from your illness – allowing it to focus on getting better.

BREATHE TO RELAX

Perhaps you feel too uneasy to relax or you can't lie still enough. Your mind races from one thought to another and everything seems to distract you. This is because your mind is trapped in a cycle of stress and one of the best ways of breaking free from it is to practise a deep breathing exercise – called rhythmic or circular breathing.

Just sit or lie in a comfortable position. Begin by exhaling all the air from your lungs. Hold for a moment, then breathe in clear, healthy oxygen into your lungs. Hold this breath, then slowly exhale, slowing down the out breath. Breathe in slowly once again

– fill your lungs to capacity. Hold it a moment. Then exhale – once again slowing down the out breath.

Continue with this deep and slow rhythmic breathing for a few minutes. Feel that you're breathing out stress and tension from your whole body.

If you do this breathing exercise a few minutes before relaxation, it will help you enter a deeper level where relaxation is more effective.

Rhythmic breathing brings your awareness to the breath; you follow it as it enters your lungs and flows back out again. Imagine your breath is like a tide coming and going, flowing on to the shore and returning to the vast ocean.

HOW TO RELAX – THE METHOD

Begin by sitting in a comfortable chair, lying down on a bed or some cushions on the floor. Take the phone off the hook. Make sure no one will disturb you for at least twenty or thirty minutes; this is your time in the day to relax and take care of yourself.

First, make yourself comfortable. Close your eyes. Become aware of all the muscles in your feet. You may wish to find the most relaxed position for your feet, so move them around. When you've done that – tighten the muscles in your feet. Hold this tension for a few moments. Release the tension and let your feet relax. Feel how your muscles are now soft, warm and relaxed. Sense how this feels. If you wish, you may repeat this exercise a number of times. Now, move your awareness to the calf muscles in your lower legs. Tense them up – keep them tight a few moments, then let them relax. Feel the tension seeping out of your calf muscles and surrounding areas.

Move your awareness to the thigh muscles in your upper legs. Tense these muscles. Hold this tightness – then let it go. Let your muscles completely relax. Feel them soft, relaxed and heavy.

Let your attention move to your hips and buttocks. Tense all the muscles in this area.

Hold this tension – then let it go. Let it relax. Feel the muscles become soft, supple and loose.

Gently move your attention to the upper and lower back muscles. Tense them up. Hold the tension for a few moments, then release this tightness. Feel a warmth spreading into your back muscles as you relax.

Move your attention to your shoulder-blades. Hold your shoulders tense for a few moments, then release the tension and feel your muscles become soft, supple and loose. Feel the tension dissolve from your shoulders.

Focus your attention to your arms and hands. Make a tight fist with your hands – hold this tension, then let it go.

Open your hands and feel the muscles in your arms relax.

Tighten your stomach muscles. Hold your muscles tight for a few moments, then breathe out all the tension from your body and nervous system.

Move to your chest. Take in a deep breath – hold it a few moments, then let it go. As you release the breath, feel all tension and stress leave your body.

Bring your awareness to your facial muscles. Begin by tensing the muscles in your forehead – as if putting a frown on your face. Tense the jaw muscles. Hold for a few seconds then let go. Feel a warm glow spreading into your face as your muscles relax.

Tense the eye muscles – just to a level that's comfortable for you. Hold them tense for a moment. Then let go and feel your eyes relax.

Be aware of your whole body now – feel how relaxed it is.

Repeat these exercises if you wish, starting with the feet and ending at the face and head. By following this sequence you open the channels of healing in your body.

CREATIVE VISUALISATION – USING THE POWER OF YOUR MIND TO HEAL YOURSELF

Once you've achieved physical relaxation, the next step is to relax your mind to a level where you can effectively heal yourself. To do this you may wish to journey in your mind to your favourite place: a place you visited as a child, a holiday you took by the sea or in the countryside. All of these images are powerful tools in helping the mind to relax.

Here's an example: picture yourself out walking along a country pathway early on a warm summer's morning. Song birds call out. The wild flowers give off their sweet fragrances. Feel yourself slowing down – becoming a part of nature – a part of this warm summer's day. As you walk along the country pathway you come to a small wooden gate, which you open, and pass through.

The path leads you down to the sea. You pause for a few moments and listen to the peaceful sounds of the waves as they flow on to the shore. It is so soothing, so peaceful.

You continue walking until you arrive at your favourite place on the beach, where you lie down and rest on the soft golden sand. Your inner being is at peace.

THE LEMON EXERCISE

This creative visualisation exercise helps to show you how powerful your mind really is.

It is a good idea to practise the lemon exercise along with relaxation. It will help you gain confidence as you tap into and influence your own healing mechanisms.

Make yourself comfortable – close your eyes and visualise a real lemon. Take the lemon in your hand. Move your hand over its wax-like surface. With your fingernails, scrape the skin of the lemon. See the spray as you penetrate the skin. Smell the beautiful aroma of lemon as the juice pours out and feel the juice between your fingers. Now place the lemon on the table, get a knife and cut the lemon in two. Pick up one half of the lemon and continue peeling back the skin with your fingers. Break a segment of lemon and put it in your mouth – taste how sour the juice is. Notice what happens.

Take another slice of lemon and put it in your mouth. Taste the juice flowing on to your tongue and swirling around your mouth. Just notice and be aware. If you've done this exercise correctly you'll notice that you've activated your saliva glands using the power of your own mind.

This opens up a range of possibilities; this ability can be used to reduce blood pressure for example, or to mobilise blood circulation within the body.

Using this technique, you can make your immune system work more effectively to heal anything from a sore throat to a broken bone, a headache to a leg ulcer.

Anne was chopping vegetables when the knife slipped. The cut was so deep that blood gushed from it like a fountain. Anne had been to see me many years before with an irritable bowel condition; she remembered some of the visualisation techniques I taught her. Calmly sitting down she visualised the image of a tap on the end of her finger. She saw herself slowly turning off the tap. Within forty seconds the bleeding stopped, but the cut was so deep it would require stitching. When Anne got to the hospital the doctors were amazed; given the nature of the wound, they said they'd never seen blood stop flowing so quickly before – without medical assistance. It was remarkable.

Once you've carried out the lemon exercise, you can focus your healing power to the area of any illness. Visualise this power as a ray of colour flowing to the problem area.

Children are great at visualisation and at times dream up funny, interesting images to help in the healing process. Some are of ray guns that wipe out the diseased part. Some imagine soldiers with hand grenades, warplanes and tanks to take out the bad guys. Some see an army of little people scrubbing clean the walls of the asthmatic lung.

It's always best to come up with your own personal healing image as it represents a more powerful meaning to your psyche. During relaxation, ask your subconscious mind to suggest an effective image to help heal your particular problem.

In his book *Mind Your Body*, Admiral E.H. Shattock describes how he used his own particular visualisation technique to cure two major conditions. The first was osteoarthritis, a degeneration of the cartilage of the hip joint. The other was a benign enlargement of the prostate gland. He managed to heal these serious conditions by first directing his white blood cells into clearing away and dissolving diseased tissue – then calling on his red blood cells to accelerate and repair the damaged parts of his body. Later on, Shattock used visualisation to overcome back strain, heal infection in the root canals of his lower jaw and dissolve a polyp in his nasal passage.

Harry, a retired pilot, was told his cancer had returned – he had to start chemotherapy right away. Having had the treatment before, Harry was told this time he was going to be very ill and was so terrified he couldn't think straight. I got him to relax and to visualise himself in a hospital bed with a drip attached to his arm.

I asked him to think of somewhere secure and special – a place he could feel safe and relaxed. Ever the pilot, Harry 'flew' above the dark clouds to golden sunshine.

I then suggested he see the image as liquid sunshine, coming through a drip into his arm, flooding his whole body with vibrant light. A smile crossed his face as he relaxed into the image.

Harry went home and told his two sons, both doctors, of his newfound technique. They urged him to be more realistic and to prepare himself for the severe sickness that would follow chemotherapy. But Harry went to the hospital each week for his 'liquid sunshine' as he now called it and left singing like a bird. The nurses and patients couldn't get over his good humour – he was a tonic for everyone, they said. The doctors were amazed at how he avoided sickness and curious as to the 'little trick' he used. His sons, too, were puzzled but admitted that whatever he'd done had worked for him.

There are many ways to visualise, to heal and improve yourself. Over the years I've helped thousands of people with various self-healing exercises. Here are some more of my favourites and I share them with you.

THE HEALING HOUSE

The following is a series of exercises based around the idea of a familiar house with healing rooms.

First make yourself comfortable. Close your eyes and focus on your breathing for a few minutes. Just allow your breathing to slow down. When you're ready, begin whatever exercise is relevant to you.

The healing room

You walk down the hallway until you come to a door with a sign saying 'The Healing Room'. You turn the door handle and walk in. The room is filled with brilliant light. In the centre of the room is a chair. You sit on this chair and a lovely feeling of peace flows over you.

In your mind you ask for healing. You become aware of hands resting gently on your head. A sensation of warmth flows through you.

You feel the presence of hands on your chest and back. Once again a feeling of warmth flows through you. You then ask for a specific healing. Almost immediately you feel hands on that very place. Healing energy flows into that whole area. Gradually the healing begins to fade – you've absorbed all the healing rays you need to nourish your whole system. Come back to the healing room any time you wish.

The medicine room

You walk down the hallway until you come to a door with a sign saying 'The Medicine Room'. You open the door and enter. It's a lovely warm bright room with your favourite colours on the walls. You immediately feel at home here. There are a number of shelves on one wall, with the most beautiful assortment of coloured bottles.

The colours range from red to orange, yellow, green, blue, violet, indigo; they're all here – a rainbow of vibrant colours. As you look closer one bottle has your name on it, written in gold letters. Instinctively you know it's the medicine you need.

You reach up and take the medicine bottle, admiring its beautiful translucent colour. You drink all the liquid that's inside the bottle. It makes you feel so good. It's exactly what you need to feel healthy and well again. Come to the medicine room any time you wish.

The energising room

You walk down the hallway until you come to a door with a sign saying 'The Energising Room'. You turn the door handle and walk in. The room feels familiar; immediately you feel at home here. Everything in the room looks bright and peaceful. You sit by the window where the sun blazes through. Shafts of light radiate through you.

You feel the warmth of these rays as they penetrate every cell of your mind and body. Your energy levels begin to rise. Your batteries are now on full power. You feel charged up and ready to go. The sunlight begins to fade. You've absorbed all the energy you need to nourish your entire system. Come back to the energising room any time you wish.

The confidence room

You walk down the hallway until you come to a door with a sign saying 'The Confidence Room'. You turn the door handle and walk in. The room feels familiar; immediately you feel at home here. Everything in the room looks bright and peaceful. In the centre of the room is a desk and a relaxing chair. On the desk is a large book. You sit at the desk and open the book. Written in the book is your

234

name in gold lettering. As you turn the pages, all the qualities you need to feel confident and secure within yourself are written down here – especially for you.

Your mind absorbs all these qualities. You can now accomplish anything in your life that was difficult before; everything seems easy. Everything seems possible. Come back to the confidence room any time you wish.

The good luck room

You walk down the hallway until you come to a door with a sign saying 'The Good Luck Room'. You turn the door handle and walk in. The whole room is gold – the walls and ceiling painted gold. The floor is covered with a beautiful gold carpet. You walk to a gold chair and sit at a beautiful gold desk. On the desk is a sea of diamonds. The diamonds are all shapes and sizes, sparkling with iridescent light and colour. You reach down and run your hands through them. Beneath the desk you notice a drawer. You open it and find it filled to capacity with gold coins. You run your hands through the coins as if through confetti. It makes you feel rich.

You say this affirmation: 'I'm now attracting wealth and good luck. Everything I touch is filled with riches.'

Immerse yourself in this feeling of abundance and wealth. Come back to the good luck room any time you wish.

The angel room

You walk down the hallway until you come to a door with a sign saying 'The Angel Room'. You turn the door handle and walk in. The room is full of burning candles – their light dances across the shadowy room. A beautiful scent fills your whole being with magic and wonder. You sit in the centre of the light of the candles and immerse yourself in a sea of golden white light.

Then a beautiful bright angel appears in front of you and touches you deep inside. Another angel appears on your right filling you with happiness. An angel appears on your left filling you with peace and love. Another appears behind you and you feel its gentle touch on your shoulders. Into their presence you relax completely.

If there's anything you wish to ask, let it form in your mind – the answer will follow. If you want help with an aspect of your life, just ask; place it gently into the hands of your angels. Come back to the angel room any time you wish.

THE HEALING POWER OF MUSIC

I frequently use music in my clinic as a tool for healing. Music quickly brings us into a meditative state and enables us to tap quickly into our self-healing powers. The benefits are enormous. Music:

- lifts the mood
- regulates our bodily systems
- puts us in touch with feelings and emotions we thought we'd forgotten
- helps to increase our imagery perception
- helps us to create the right mood to visualise
- enhances creativity
- acts as a natural tranquilliser
- promotes a good night's sleep
- helps us take our minds off our problems
- transports us to a time when we felt happy in ourselves.

Some pieces of music I find particularly beneficial are:

- 'The Fairy Ring', 'The Brighter Side' and 'Silver Wings' by Mike Rowland
- 'River of Life' by Fredrik Karlsson
- 'Lazaris Remembers Lemuria' by David Frank and Steven Boone

※ 'Dance of the Blessed Spirits' by Christophe von Gluck
※ 'Largo Ma Non Tanto' by J.S. Bach
※ 'Canon' by Johann Pachelbel.

Put on a piece of music – whichever you find most relaxing. Check the volume level so that it's just right. Then make yourself comfortable. Close your eyes and listen to the music. Let it pour into you. Breathe it in. Feel it flow into every pore of your body. Let your mind settle.

Release any thoughts or images of stress, worry or anxiety. See them being washed away by the music.

Let the music vibrate into your entire being. Soak it in for twenty or thirty minutes.

COLOUR HEALING

This exercise is wonderful for strengthening your inner being by clearing negative influences from your energy fields.

Close your eyes and relax your whole body. Focus your mind on your breathing. Let your breath and your mind slow down.

※ Breathe the colour red into your body. Imagine your aura and body filling with the colour red.

※ Change the colour red to orange. As you breathe in, see your body filling up with the colour orange.

※ Change the colour orange to yellow. As you breathe in, see your body filling up with the colour yellow.

※ Change the colour yellow to green. As you breathe in, see your body filling up with the colour green.

※ Change the colour green to blue. As you breathe in, see your body filling up with the colour blue.

※ Change the colour blue to violet. As you breathe in, see your body filling up with the colour violet.

❧ Change the colour violet to white. As you breathe in, see your whole body filling up with the colour white.

HOW TO CONTROL PAIN

If you ask a person who's experiencing pain what colour they imagine pain to be – most likely they'd say the colour red. You can use this colour in a very good visualisation technique to help control pain. First, enter the relaxation level and visualise your pain as deep red. Imagine the redness changing to orange; hold this image for a few moments. Now change the orange colour to yellow. Then to green, the colour of nature. Change from green to cool blue. Sense the pain getting less and less as you change colour. Finally, visualise the whole area completely blue, like a deep sea blue.

Do this exercise as often as you like throughout the day.

You could also try placing something blue over the painful area, such as a blue cloth or scarf or a blue towel. If the pain is in your foot, for example, you could wear a blue sock.

HOW TO STOP WORRYING

My favourite exercise for worry is the balloon exercise. Many people have written to tell me how this simple exercise has helped them deal successfully with a particular worry or problem.

First begin with relaxation. Imagine you're out in the countryside; see yourself surrounded by nature. The sky is clear blue. Birds are singing. Inhale the scent from your favourite flowers. Now, visualise yourself writing down on some pieces of paper all your worries, all your innermost negative thoughts and feelings. Make a parcel of each worry – big parcels for the larger worries and small ones for the minor ones. Tie coloured ribbons around the parcels if you like.

Then visualise a big, brightly coloured balloon attached to a large basket. It's tied by ropes to a fence or gate near you.

You place all your worry parcels in the basket. Then untie the rope and watch as the balloon climbs higher and higher into the clear blue sky, until it's just a dot on the horizon. Watch it as it disappears, vanishing for good with all your worries in it. You feel lighter and brighter – free to enjoy life again. You can do this exercise any time you feel troubled or worried about something.

POSITIVE AFFIRMATIONS

Affirmations can have a strong influence on our health, happiness and in our daily lives. Each thought and word is like a statement or declaration – either positive or negative. When we say, 'I don't feel well', we're effectively reciting an affirmation that creates a negative feeling. Feelings always follow thought. We think the thought, and the feeling follows.

Therefore, if we think good thoughts we experience good feelings. Consequently, if we think a bad or negative thought, the feeling and effect (no matter how subtle) follows.

If negative thoughts are continually focused upon, a negative pattern emerges and we experience this negativity in our daily lives. Some see the bottle half-full, while others see it half-empty. It's all a matter of perception.

Positive thinking opens up new possibilities, while negative thinking shuts off the possibility of anything good happening. A simple shift in consciousness from 'I can't' to 'I can' makes a whole world of difference to any situation. You simply drop the 't'. Any time you catch yourself saying 'I can't find a way out of this problem' – learn to drop the 't. You can then look at your problem with new eyes.

Say, 'I can – I can, I can' as many times as you wish during the day and a whole world of new possibilities will open up for you.

Emile Coué lived in France from 1857 to 1926. A chemist for thirty years, he became interested in the mind's power to heal the body. Coué developed a system called 'auto-suggestion' – another term for affirmations. His famous and often-quoted saying is 'Every day in every way, I'm getting better and better'. In his book on auto-suggestion he says, 'Every thought entirely filling our mind becomes true for us and tends to transform itself into action.'

Affirmations can be said in as many interesting and creative ways as you can imagine:

- You can say them aloud to yourself or in a whisper.
- You can even sing your affirmations while going around the house.
- Write them a number of times in your notebook or diary.
- Draw your affirmations with crayons and pin them to your bedroom wall – they are there when you sleep and when you wake.
- You can say your affirmations while walking along or doing exercises.

I was giving a lecture one evening on positive thinking and self-healing in a children's school, and couldn't help but notice brightly coloured drawings adorning the walls of the classroom. They were crayon drawings of rainbows and flowers, and over each one in bright colours were the words: 'We are special'. The paintings were everywhere, some with variations, but the message was still the same: 'We are special'. What a powerful message to give to children, I thought. But where, oh where was the message for adults?

So, adults! Why not write out your own affirmations, or draw a picture and paste it on your wall.

Affirmations should be repeated, over and over again, to help dissolve the old negative thought patterns that may have been lying in your consciousness for years. Each time you practise an affirmation exercise, I suggest you repeat it at least thirty times and recite it in the present tense. Here's an example:

I'm now happy, healthy and full of vibrant energy.

I'm now leaving the past behind. I'm open and receptive for good experiences to come into my life.

My knee is now healing (or whatever body part is affected).

Healing energy flows through me, washing all disease from my body.

Creative and inspiring ideas flow easily into my mind.

I relax with every breath I take.

Each day my health is getting better and better.

My ability to concentrate is becoming stronger.

I communicate effectively with everyone I come into contact with.

Infinite, abundant riches are flowing into my life.

The subconscious doesn't have a sense of humour; positive or negative it gives us what we ask. Some typical negative affirmations are 'I can't remember the name of that person I met five minutes ago. My memory seems to be getting worse – I can't even remember what I did yesterday.'

If you keep telling yourself your memory is getting worse – it will. The flip side of this is the positive affirmation, 'My memory is always good, it serves me well.' If you repeat this often, soon you will notice how your memory improves.

When you practise positive affirmations, you quickly become aware how many negative words and sentences you use, even within the space of five minutes.

When I first started to write this book, I was consumed with negativity, morning, noon and night. I just felt I wasn't good enough for the task. My mind kept saying, 'I can't type. Can't use a word processor. I've never written a book before.'

All this negativity kept running around and around in my head. 'If only I'd listened to my teacher at school more. If only I'd done a course in creative writing. If only! If only!'

Limitations in your mind are like traffic lights permanently on red. When you learn to think positively and move forward, you change the traffic lights from red to green. There are thousands of possibilities waiting for us as we awake each morning, so make a decision now to paint only happy pictures in your mind.

LAUGHTER – THE BEST MEDICINE

Laughter has such a powerful effect on our health. If I can get a patient to laugh, the effect on their energy field is amazing as I watch it free out and expand. When practising this self-healing programme I encourage you to have at least four good belly-laughs a day.

Laughter releases us from isolation and depression. It causes our immune system to work more effectively. It helps lighten the mood and the thoughts, enabling us to see our problems in a totally new light.

In his book *Anatomy of an Illness*, Norman Cousins explains how he developed a serious illness called 'ankylosing spondylitis' – the connective tissue in his spine was disintegrating. He could no longer move his limbs, his joints seized up and were extremely painful, so that turning over in bed was an ordeal. Specialists told him that they'd never witnessed a recovery – the chances were one in five hundred. Cousins says: 'If I was going to be that one in five hundred, I had better be something more than a passive observer!' He began to pore over books, concluding that positive emotions might produce positive effects on the body's chemistry. With his doctors' help, he checked himself out of hospital into a hotel.

Cousins took large doses of vitamin C as a substitute for the many tablets he had been taking for his condition. He developed a 'programme of laughter' and watched tapes of *Candid Camera* and Marks brothers movies, remarking that: 'Ten minutes of genuine belly laughing had an anaesthetic effect and gave me at least two hours of pain-free sleep.' He made a complete recovery and went back to playing tennis, golf and horse-riding.

WRITE OUT YOUR PROBLEMS

Another self-healing method I strongly recommend is to write out your problems every day. Keep a workbook and in it you can safely release a lot of harmful stress, fears, worries and anxieties from your mind and body. Write everything down. When you've finished, turn the page and then write out possible solutions (if any) to your problems, and what actions you can take to solve them. Remember that by simply writing down your problems you've already taken action.

If you do this correctly, you'll be surprised what changes it quickly brings to your mind, your body and to your life.

The daily habit of writing out your problems helps get rid of the negativity that has accumulated in your system. Your mind is then open and clear to receive bright creative ideas and possible solutions.

HOW TO DO HANDS-ON HEALING

It is always best to practise healing first on your own family. This acts as a good safeguard from picking up any negative energies that you may not be able to handle. First, shake your hands gently to get the energy flowing through them. Then bring the palms of your hands a few inches apart from each other. Move them gently away, then bring them close. Do this a few times and see what you feel.

With a bit of practice you will feel a ball of energy between both hands. You may experience the healing energy as a mild tingling sensation, a hot or a cool feeling.

Now you are ready to try it out. Ask your partner, child or even your pet cat or dog to sit still. Bring your hands a few inches from their body. See, can you feel their aura? Move your hands gently about an inch from their body. Then intuitively sense where you need to place your hands. Leave them there for as long as it takes and feel this healing power flow from your hands through them.

When you have finished take your hands gently away and give them a shake.

Well how did you do? Ask for feedback if you can. You did it!

HOW TO DO ABSENT HEALING

You should also practise absent healing with a family member or a family pet at first. Relax and focus on your breathing for a while. Then bring up a picture of them in your mind and visualise a white light going to them.

Take as long as you need, then see them happy, in good health and surrounded in this white light.

In your heart what would be your greatest wish for them? Hold that thought. When you are ready gently break contact in your mind and come back to yourself.

MY WISH FOR YOU

I was born chronically ill and nearly died. The caul had protected me and saved my life. As I struggled to breathe, Granny Brien threw her warm arms around me and enveloped me in her love. She helped me to breathe, to live, to find myself in the world. Later, when I was without hope, I was rescued by my spirit friends – a shimmering light, a calming voice, through a troubled night.

I was close to death, but also to life. My spirit friends were helping me, showing me the way, preparing me for a life of healing. This was my path and my journey – to overcome my illness and develop my healing gift, so that I might help others.

Throughout my journey many people have come to me, alone in their illness, their heartache and pain. I've seen them transformed; a blissful face as the pain subsides, tears of joy as a burden is eased, springtime as their darkness drifts away. All of these wonderful people have told their stories so that others may find comfort and peace. Knowing them has deepened and expanded my experience of life. I hope they have enriched yours too, and inspired you on your path.

May my gift of healing be a blessing to you, and may it bring you health, happiness and joy. May it nourish your beautiful spirit, and make it shine ever brighter.

BIBLIOGRAPHY

Coué, Emile, *Self Mastery Through Conscious Autosuggestion*, George Allen & Unwin Ltd, London, 1922

Coué, Emile, *The Practice of Autosuggestion*, George Allen & Unwin Ltd, London, 1922

Cousins, Norman, *Anatomy of an Illness – As Perceived by the Patient*, Bantam Books, London, 1987

Edwards, Harry, *A Guide to the Understanding and Practice of Spiritual Healing*, The Healer Publishing Company Limited, 1974

Sechrist, Elsie, *Auras*, A.R.E. Press, Virginia Beach, 1964

Shattock, E H, *Mind Your Body – A Practical Method of Self-healing*, Turnstone Press, Wellingborough, 1979

BORN TO HEAL –
THE INVISIBLE WORLD

A documentary portrait of an Irish Spiritual Healer

This unique documentary tells the compelling story of Tony Hogan from his birth to the present day, showing him as a young man developing his ability to heal.

We hear amazing stories of people being healed and, for the first time, we see live footage of Auras – the human energy fields of men, women and children being transformed by Tony's healing hands. We also see Tony use his other extraordinary ability – that of Absent Healing.

This beautifully-crafted film touches the heart of who we really are. It will open your perception to another world – the world you always knew was there – the spirit world, making this a treasured film that you will want to see over and over again.

The film is narrated by English actor John Nettles and beautifully photographed by Cathal Black, the gifted filmmaker who gave us 'Korea' and 'Love and Rage'.

Running Time: 54 mins. VHS/NTSC.
Price: 25 Euro includes P&P

Contact: Cathal Black Films, 161 Monalea Grove, Firhouse, Dublin 24, Ireland or e-mail: forge@indigo.ie